"I always knew that you could cook anything and make it healthier and my mum seemed to be able to do this. You've not only shown me how and helped me lose weight, but helped me become a better cook!"

MARY JANE WRIGHT

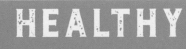

"...en like ...t so ...spiration and encouragement."

JULIE MURDOCH

HEALTHY

"I love Pinch of Nom. My favourite recipe is Lemon Chicken (minus the pineapple), which makes it exactly the same as a takeaway. PoN have opened my world to eating differently."

IRENE MASON

"Pinch of Nom has given me loads of fab ideas to cook, not just for my partner and I who are dieting, but also for my son who is losing weight and LOVING the food in the process."

EMMA BUCKMASTER

"Brilliant, easy-to-follow recipes. I love PoN, makes cooking quick and simple ... so many diverse recipes to choose from."

CHRISTINE DAVIS

"Without PoN I would be 33 pounds heavier no question. You guys and this site are my inspiration. Thank you so much."

LINDA MCCARTHUR

"Absolutely awesome at inspiring me to keep going! A diet with boring food is impossible and this site gives you so many tasty ideas for food! Love, love, love it."

LAURA OLIVER

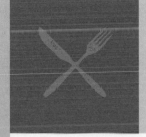

"Great site! Has helped me understand the importance of vegetables in my diet and the effect they can have on weight loss."

ANN HORSMAN

"We love Pinch of Nom in our house. Hubby isn't even on a diet and loves the recipes."

LAURA DENNIS

"Brilliant, easy-to-follow recipes that help me feel like I don't have to miss out."

LENA BARKSBY

BRILLIANT

"My favourite recipe is Lamb Rogan Josh – I just hated giving up my spicy food because of the calories. Pinch of Nom was a revelation when I discovered it."

DENISE ALEXANDER

"Healthy menus that actually look/taste like they're not on a diet and that my teenagers want to eat!"

CLAIRE ARMSTRONG

AWESOME & INSPIRING

Pinch

OF

Nom

For CATH

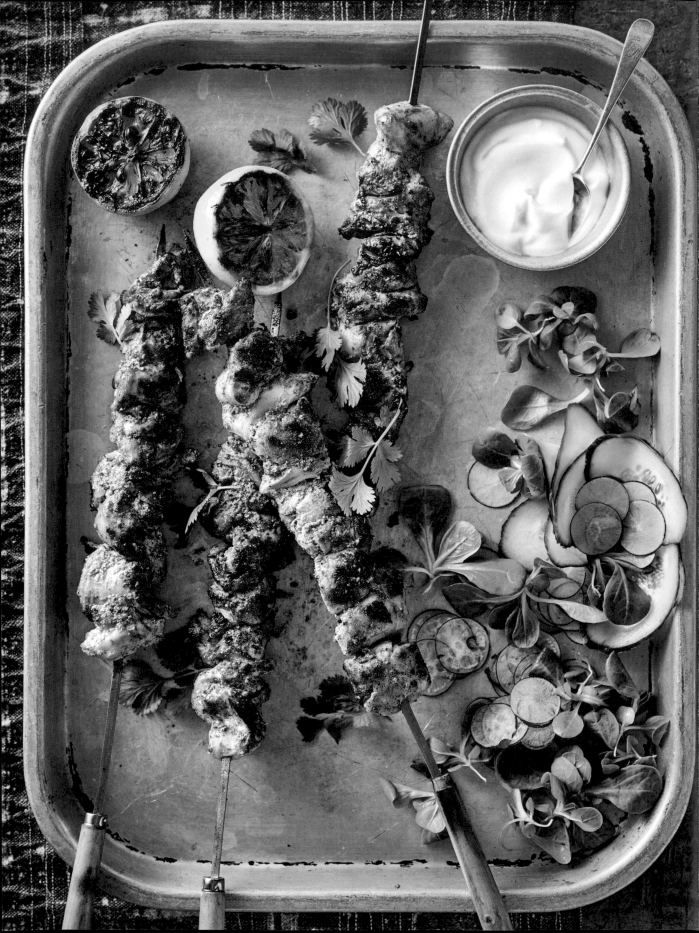

KATE ALLINSON & KAY FEATHERSTONE

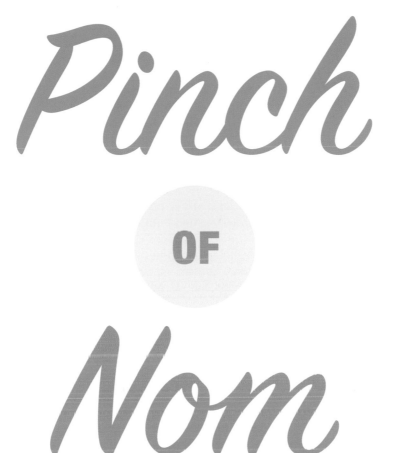

Pinch of Nom

100 HOME-STYLE RECIPES FOR HEALTH AND WEIGHT LOSS

ST. MARTIN'S
ESSENTIALS

NEW YORK

First published in the United States by St. Martin's Essentials,
an imprint of St. Martin's Publishing Group

PINCH OF NOM. Copyright © 2019 by Kate Allinson and Kay Featherstone.
Photographs copyright © 2019 by Mike English. All rights reserved. Printed in Germany.
For information, address St. Martin's Publishing Group, 120 Broadway, New York, NY 10271.

www.stmartins.com

Art Direction, Design, and Illustration: Emma Wells, Nic&Lou Design
Food Styling: Kate Wesson
Prop Styling: Cynthia Blackett

The Library of Congress Cataloging-in-Publication Data is available upon request.

ISBN 978-1-250-26955-3 (paper over board)
ISBN 978-1-250-26956-0 (ebook)

Our books may be purchased in bulk for promotional, educational,
or business use. Please contact your local bookseller or the Macmillan Corporate
and Premium Sales Department at 1-800-221-7945, extension 5442, or by email at
MacmillanSpecialMarkets@macmillan.com.

Originally published in the United Kingdom by Bluebird, an imprint of Pan Macmillan

First U.S. Edition: April 2020

10 9 8 7 6 5 4 3 2 1

Contents

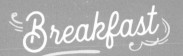
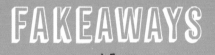
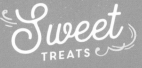

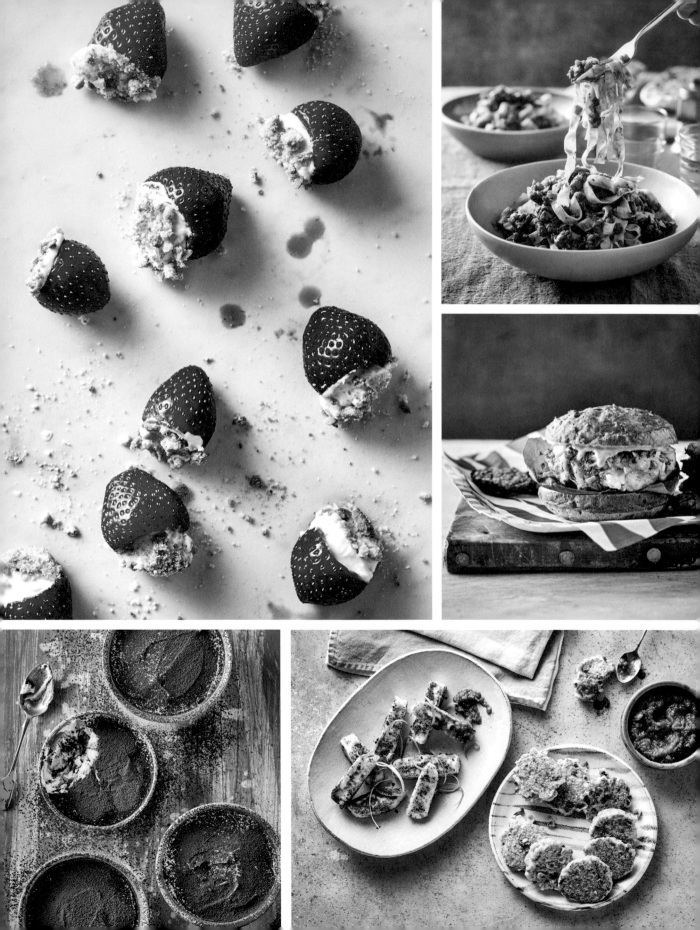

WELCOME TO

Pinch OF *Nom*

Pinch of Nom started out a few years ago over a cup of tea at the kitchen table. After a decade of working in the restaurant world, we wanted to create a place where we could share our recipes. Now we have a community of over 1.5 million using the site to find easy recipes and enjoy slimming, delicious food. And we're loving every moment!

Back when we were working long shifts in a high-pressured restaurant kitchen, it was always easiest to grab unhealthy food on the go. Eventually the time came when we both needed to lose weight, so we decided to join a local weight-loss group. Immediately we noticed a lack of easy and delicious recipe ideas – and it was the same online. We were so surprised by how many people were relying on expensive "low-cal" ready-meals, lacking in flavour and variety.

One day Kate disappeared into the kitchen and came back with cheesecake-stuffed strawberries. So delicious and portable, they were a huge hit with our weight-loss group. After sharing a few more recipes with friends to great success, we had a small idea. What if we put our recipes onto a website and shared them with others? Our mission became to create easy, healthy and tasty dishes for ordinary people to enjoy.

We were amazed at how many people started to visit. Within around 6 months the website was drawing in over sixty thousand people a month. The tiny idea had become big. Bigger than we had ever imagined.

" PINCH OF NOM IS FAR BIGGER THAN WE EVER IMAGINED "

Suddenly, people were starting to lose weight. The Pinch of Nom Facebook group was growing at a rate no one had foreseen. As the group grew, it became apparent that many people who had not yet reached their goal weight and who jumped on and off the "weight-loss wagon" felt neglected by the large diet industry companies. Soon others volunteered to join us to form the Pinch of Nom team, and we started to create a space where those who were still on their journey (like us) were just as important as those who had reached their destination.

The aim of this book is to provide delicious, light recipes that don't feel like diet food. If you slip off the wagon, we want to make you feel as if climbing back on isn't so hard! You might put the book down occasionally, but it'll be just as easy to pick it right back up again.

Pinch of Nom is now much bigger than the two of us, both in terms of the team that runs it and the community that has grown from it. We are continually blown away by all the support and the love that feeds through that community on a daily basis.

This book wouldn't have existed without every single member of our Facebook group, every visitor to the website and every person who has contributed to Pinch of Nom: team members, volunteers, taste testers and commenters that have provided constructive criticism to improve the recipes and content on the site.

This book is for you. We hope you love cooking the recipes as much as we've loved putting this all together.

Kate and Kay x

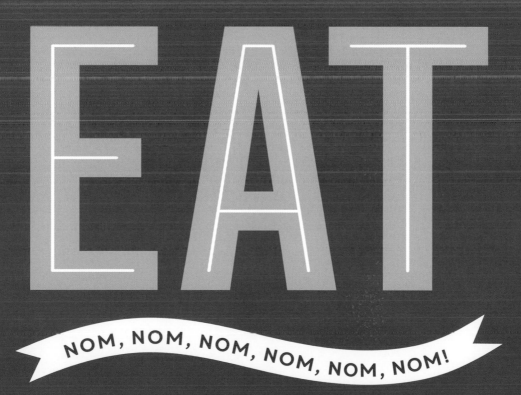

Healthy
RECIPES
that we all want to
EAT

NOM, NOM, NOM, NOM, NOM, NOM, NOM!

The FOOD

HEALTHY RECIPES *that* DON'T TASTE LIKE DIET FOOD

As a classically trained chef, Kate has always looked at recipes and dishes, then worked out how to improve or re-create them. We've worked together on transforming some of our favourite dishes into healthy indulgences – including turning high-calorie takeaways into "fakeaways" that are even tastier than their calorific counterparts.

Switching out a few key ingredients has a massive impact on the calorie, fat or sugar content of food. It tastes just as delicious – especially when flavours are enhanced with clever spicing and seasoning.

22 ALL-TIME FAVOURITES *and* 80 BRAND-NEW RECIPES

We have included our most popular recipes from the website in this book, as it wouldn't be a Pinch of Nom book without them! The rest of the recipes are brand-new labours of love that we hope you love as much as we do.

QUICK, UNPRETENTIOUS FOOD

You can prepare most of the recipes in this book in under 30 minutes. It was important to the Pinch of Nom team that the recipes were easily accessible and so we've used ingredients that you can use time and again to save on cost. So many chefs forget that we don't all have a pinch of white truffle at home! We only use less familiar ingredients where they add a unique touch to the dish – and we've tried to include them more than once, so you don't have a pile of dusty ingredients at the back of the cupboard.

DEVELOPED *and* TESTED *in* PINCH OF NOM HOME KITCHENS

Early on in the Pinch of Nom history, we decided that our recipes should always be authentic. With so many untested "diet" recipes floating around using stock photography, we decided that every recipe should be made, tested and photographed without artistic licence, which is the approach we've used for the cookbook.

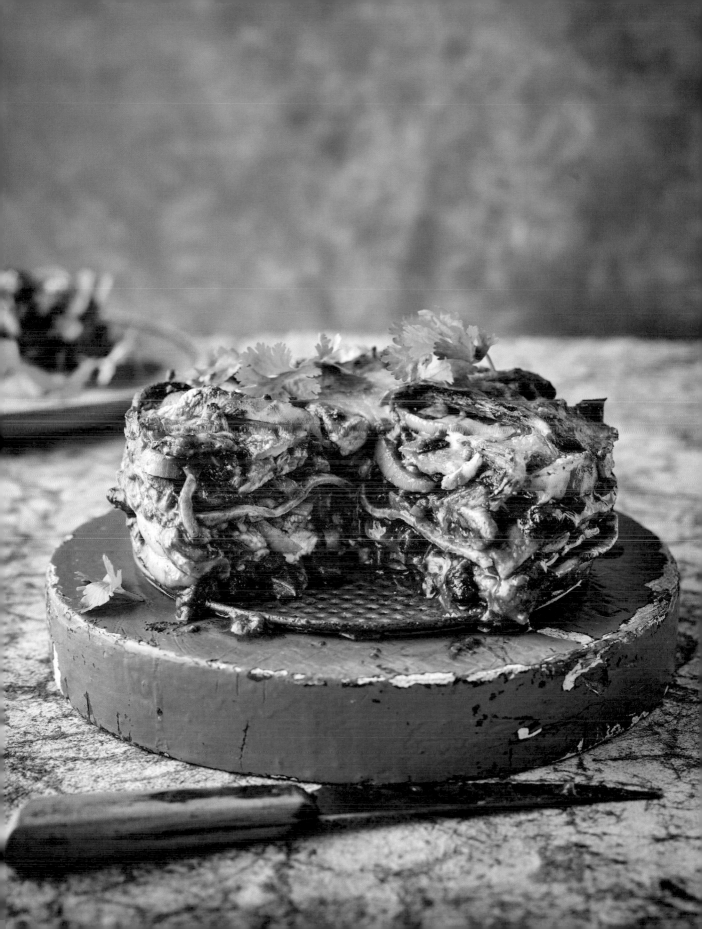

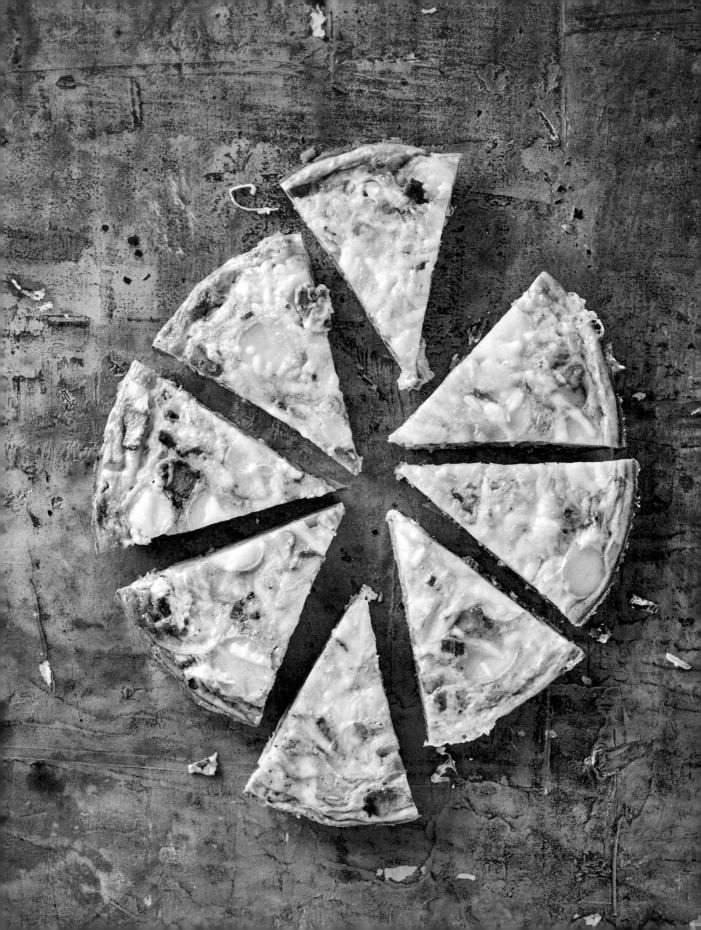

How Our RECIPES WORK

EVERYDAY LIGHT

At Pinch of Nom, we believe in the ethos of "everything in moderation." With this in mind, our **Everyday Light** recipes are those you can have at any time: they're easy on the calories, filling and perfect for every day. You may notice some of these recipes are higher in calories than those in the other categories. The reason for this is that some calories are "used up" on vegetables and other ingredients that conform to zero-point-style foods applicable to the UK's most popular diet programmes.

WEEKLY INDULGENCE

These are recipes you can add to your weekly meal plans but have one or two ingredients that make them slightly more indulgent, so should be used in moderation. A good basis of any diet should be that you don't have to miss out on enjoying dinner parties or the odd treat here or there.

SPECIAL OCCASION

Our **Special Occasion** recipes have your back! Lower in calories than regular desserts, snacks or treats, this section still comes out tops against high-calorie versions. However, the aforementioned ethos of "everything in moderation" should come to mind with these. Save these recipes for pushing the boat out and for ... you guessed it ... special occasions!

CALORIES AND VALUES

Our calorie counts are all worked out per individual serving. This does not include accompaniments for specific recipes, such as rice or potatoes. This is because we give these notes as a serving suggestion only. You can easily swap out rice and pasta for veggie low-calorie alternatives, such as cauliflower rice.

We have not included "values" from mainstream diet programmes as these are everchanging and we want this book to be a resource that is always up to date.

OUR RECIPE ICONS

 Suitable for vegetarians

 Suitable for freezing
For all freezer-friendly recipes, we recommend defrosting completely before heating until piping hot.

GF Suitable for those following a gluten-free diet

TASTE TESTED

Over the last few months, a group of two hundred Pinch of Nom fans have been huddled together in a secret Facebook group. Each recipe has been tested by twenty people, all submitting feedback and suggestions for development.

This process has been essential in the creation of this book and we want to extend a huge thank-you to these members for their invaluable input. (You can find their names in the back of the book.)

KEY INGREDIENTS

PROTEIN

Lean meats are a great source of protein, providing essential nutrients and fantastic filling power. In all recipes with meat as an ingredient, make sure you use the leanest cuts and trim off all visible fat. Fish is another great source of protein and naturally low in fat. One of our favourite phrases is: "if it swims, it slims!" Fish provides nutrients that the body struggles to produce naturally, making it perfect for some of Pinch of Nom's super-slimming recipes. One-third of the recipes in the book are veggie, but you can always use vegetarian protein options instead of meat in our recipes.

LOW-FAT DAIRY

Swapping in clever alternatives for high-fat dairy products can instantly make a dish healthier. We often substitute low-fat soft cheese or yogurt for higher-fat ingredients.

TINS

Don't be afraid to bulk buy some of those tinned essentials! Beans, tomatoes, sweet corn … You'll find you can add many of these ingredients into Pinch of Nom stews and salads. They keep the cost of dishes down and, compared to fresh, it makes little or no difference to the flavour.

FROZEN VEG

Similarly, frozen vegetables bulk out dishes and are great low-cost alternatives for recipes like stews, where fresh options aren't necessarily required.

HERBS *and* SPICES

Pinch of Nom love a bit of spice! When you're changing ingredients for lower fat/sugar/calorie versions, one of the best ways to keep your food interesting is to season well with herbs and spices. In particular, mixed spice blends are perfect for lots of recipes in this book. Don't be shy with spices – not all of them burn your mouth off! We use garlic granules in a lot of our recipes because they are a convenient and cheaper alternative to fresh garlic and in slow cooks and stews, for example, you won't be able to tell the difference.

STOCK POTS *and* STOCK CUBES

One of Pinch of Nom's favourite ingredients is the lowly stock pot. (In the United States, Knorr markets this as "concentrated stock"– it comes in little plastic cups.) It adds instant flavour and is so versatile. Pinch of Nom use various flavoured pots throughout this book, but they are all interchangeable. Stock (bouillon) cubes can be substituted for stock pots. Red and white wine stock pots add an amazing depth to a recipe, without the calories of wine.

VINEGARS

Taste is all about balance. When you remove fat from a dish, flavours can dwindle. Most people simply make something spicy to counteract the lack of fat flavours, but the level of acidity in a dish is also really important. Poulet au Vinaigre (see page 146), for example, is a recipe that really showcases the rich, deep flavours that a good vinegar can bring to a balanced dish.

LEMONS *and* LIMES

Citrus fruits pack an absolute punch when it comes to flavour. They're perfect for adding to recipes that need an extra bit of "zing" like the Cold Asian Noodle Salad (see page 116).

TORTILLA WRAPS

Wraps are a fantastic, versatile ingredient. To add a bit of fibre and some more filling power, whole-wheat and whole-grain options are always a good choice. Pinch of Nom recipes are synonymous with creating some magic with wraps! You'll be surprised at the crazy dishes you can re-create using a lowly tortilla wrap – you can even use it in place of pastry!

WHOLE-GRAIN BREAD

A great source of fibre providing that all-important filling power, whole-grain bread can be used as it is, or broken down into breadcrumbs to make coatings for meat or Scotch eggs (Tuna Scotch Eggs, page 230).

PULSES, RICE *and* BEANS

High in both protein and fibre, tins of beans and pulses are perfect in the cupboard staples. Rice is really satisfying and, when flavoured with spices and/or seasoning, it's a great accompaniment to many of our recipes.

OATS

These are a Pinch of Nom staple. A fantastic and cost-effective ingredient, try them in our Carrot Cake Overnight Oats (see page 44). Ground down to a flour, they also make a super-filling ingredient that you can use in place of white flour.

EGGS

Protein-rich, filling, tasty and versatile, eggs are the ultimate in slimming yet satisfying ingredients. You can use them as a butter alternative for something like Lazy Mash (see page 212), or as a great source of protein for meals like our Shakshuka (see page 106). You'll always want a box in the house.

LOW-CALORIE SPRAY

One of the best ways to cut down on cooking with oils and fats is to use a low-calorie spray. It makes little difference to the way that most ingredients are cooked, but it has a huge impact on the calories because you need so much less than you would when pouring oil into a pan. You can also use olive oil spray – just be careful how much you're spraying to save calories.

SWEETENER

Some of our recipes use sweetener. We use it sparingly, but you're welcome to add less or a little more to recipes; it's all down to individual taste. You can also use natural alternatives, such as stevia or agave, but be mindful that the calorie count may change with these products.

GLUTEN-FREE BREADS

We use gluten-free ciabattas in a few of our recipes. Generally lower in calories, they also have a high fibre-density, which is a perfect way to balance your diet when you're following a low-calorie diet. They also tend to be packaged part-baked and keep for a good time at ambient temperature – which is great to reduce waste if you change your meal plans at the last minute, because they'll keep for next time!

ESSENTIAL KIT

NON-STICK PANS

If there's one bit of kit that we'd recommend, it's a decent set of non-stick pans. The better the non-stick quality of your pans, the less cooking oils and fats you will need to avoid food sticking to your pan and burning. Keep your pans in good health too – clean them properly and gently with soapy water.

MEASURING SPOONS

Want to make sure you're not putting a tablespoon of chile powder in your dish, rather than half a teaspoon? This is one of the most helpful items of kitchenware you'll ever own. Especially vital if you've ever made the aforementioned mistake, as we have never done. Never.

SPATULA

Do you need a description of a spatula? Just know that it's an essential bit of kit … If you don't own one, you should! You'll be surprised what you end up using it for. Even smacking hands away from cooling Pinch of Nom bakes, such as the Bakewell Tarts (see page 244).

FOOD PROCESSOR / BLENDER / STICK BLENDER

Many of our recipes involve making delicious, flavourful sauces from scratch, so a decent blender or food processor is a godsend! You can also use a stick blender on most occasions if you're looking for something a bit cheaper or more compact.

FINE GRATER

Using a fine grater is one of those surprising revelations. You won't believe the difference in grating cheese with a fine grater versus a standard grater. Around 1 ounce of cheese, for example, can easily cover an oven dish when using a fine grater. It's much easier to keep calories down and make your cheese go much further!

KNIFE SHARPENER

There is nothing worse than trying to chop a butternut squash up with a spoon. So why would you re-create the experience with your knives? Keep those babies sharp! It will save you so much time and effort.

TUPPERWARE *and* PLASTIC TUBS

Most of the recipes in this book are freezable and perfect for batch-cooking. It is so much easier to plan ahead when you can cook ahead too, so invest in some decent freezerproof tubs for storage.

RAMEKINS

Helping to keep portion sizes in control, ramekins are always good for desserts and bakes.

OVEN TRAYS *and* SPRINGFORM TINS

Keep these in good condition for longer by lining them with parchment paper or foil. You'll need a springform pan in our Chicken Fajita Pie (see page 74) and while it's only one recipe, this is one you'll want to make again and again – trust us!

POTATO MASHER

Used in a variety of recipes, you'll need a decent masher to ensure you're not straining muscles every time you want a bit of mash!

SLOW COOKER / PRESSURE COOKER

These are more of an optional favourite than essential, but we absolutely love them. Just throw in your ingredients and leave it: how easy is that? Electric pressure cookers and slow cookers are perfect for quick family meals that are made without having to stand over a cooker. Also, don't be fooled into thinking that you have to buy expensive cuts of meat for the best results. Cheaper cuts of meat often end up being tastier and more tender when slow or pressure cooking, which is a bonus for flavour and for your wallet! Many of our recipes, including the Lamb Guvech (see page 153), include methods for using a slow cooker or a pressure cooker, but we've also included traditional methods in case you don't have one.

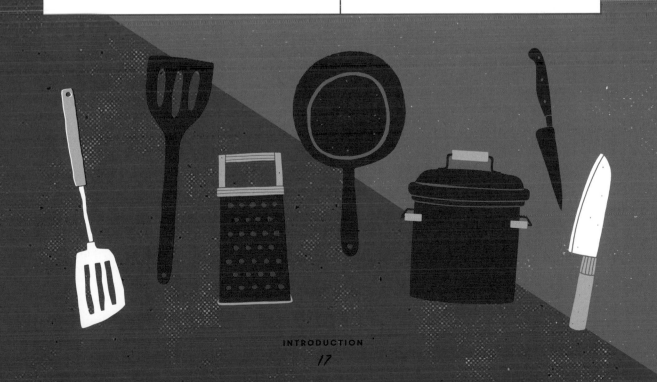

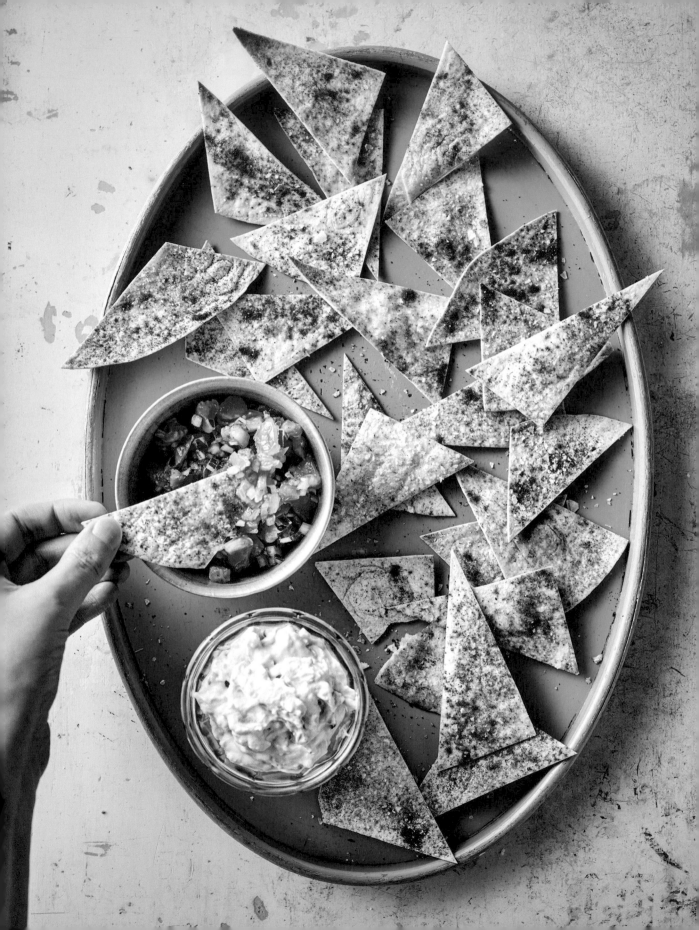

RECIPES
that work
EVERY
single time

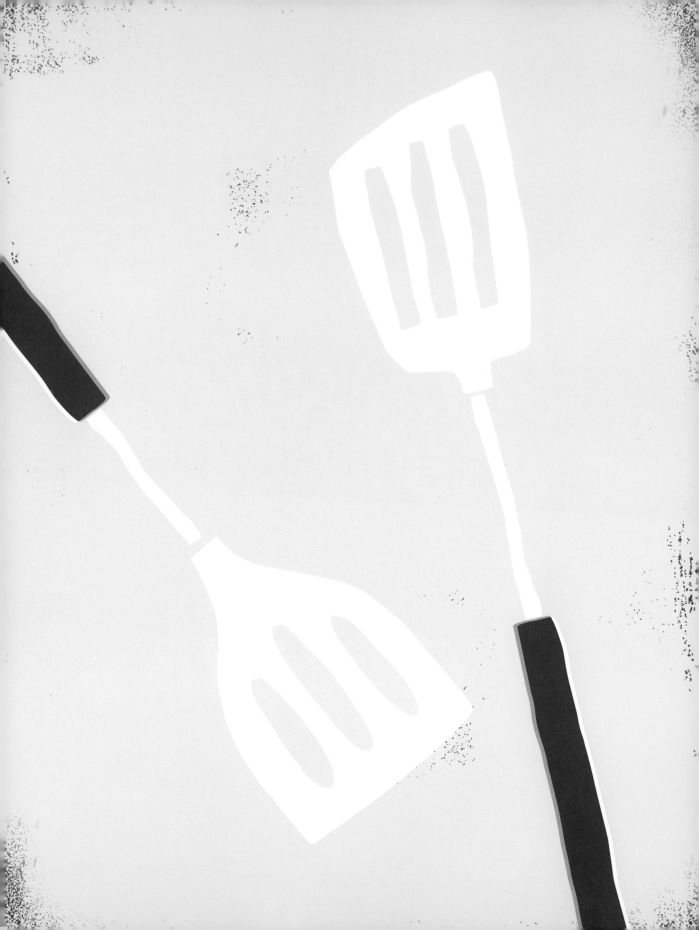

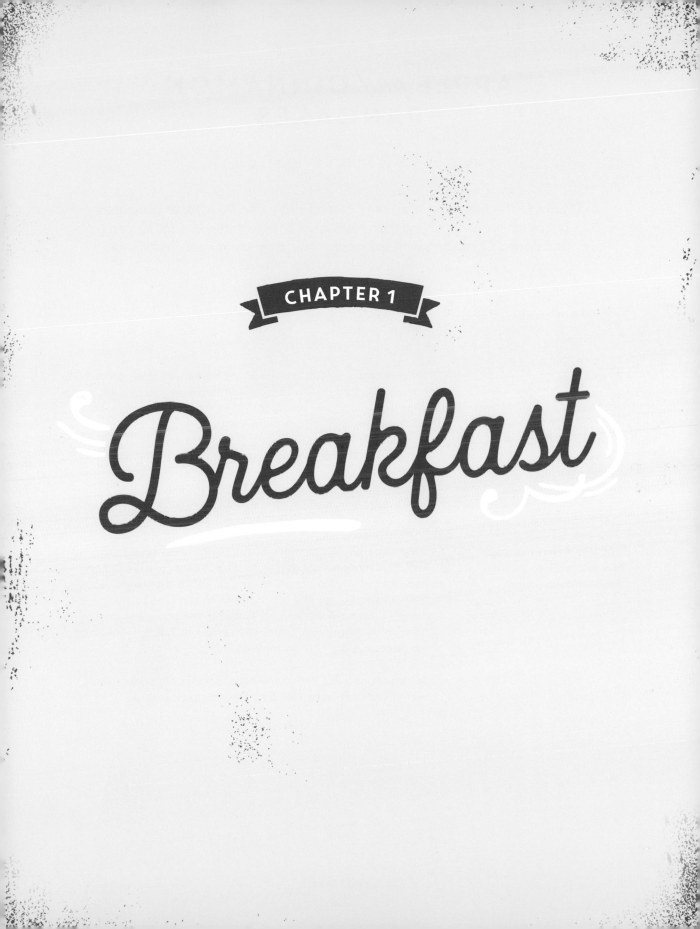

CHAPTER 1

Breakfast

APPLE *and* CINNAMON PANCAKES

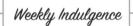

🕐 **10 MINS** | 🍲 **10 MINS** | 🔥 **341 CALS** PER SERVING

Thanks to the filling power of oats, blitzed into a fine flour, these pancakes
are much more satisfying than traditional ones, yet they are far lighter
in calories. Combined with spices and fruit, they are a really indulgent
and delicious way to start the day.

Weekly Indulgence

SERVES 1

½ cup rolled oats
1½ apples, 1 grated, ½ sliced to serve
3½ tbsp skim milk
¼ tsp ground cinnamon
1 tsp granulated sweetener, plus an
    extra pinch
2 medium eggs, beaten
2 tbsp fat-free natural yogurt
low-calorie cooking spray
fresh berries, to garnish

Blitz the oats in a food processor or blender until finely ground (like
a flour). Tip into a bowl and mix in ⅓ cup of the grated apple,
along with the milk, cinnamon, ½ tsp sweetener and beaten
eggs. Set aside.

Mix the yogurt in a bowl with the remaining grated apple and a
pinch of sweetener.

Spray a large frying pan with some low-calorie cooking spray
and place it over a medium heat.

Spoon four equal quantities of the pancake batter into the hot
pan, making sure they don't touch each other (you may need to
cook them in two batches if your pan isn't big enough). Cook
for 1–2 minutes until the top starts to set and the bottom is a
golden brown colour, then carefully flip the pancakes and cook
for another few minutes, or until the bottom has coloured and
the pancakes are cooked through.

Serve the pancakes with some fresh sliced apple, some fresh
berries such as blueberries, and the grated apple and yogurt mix.

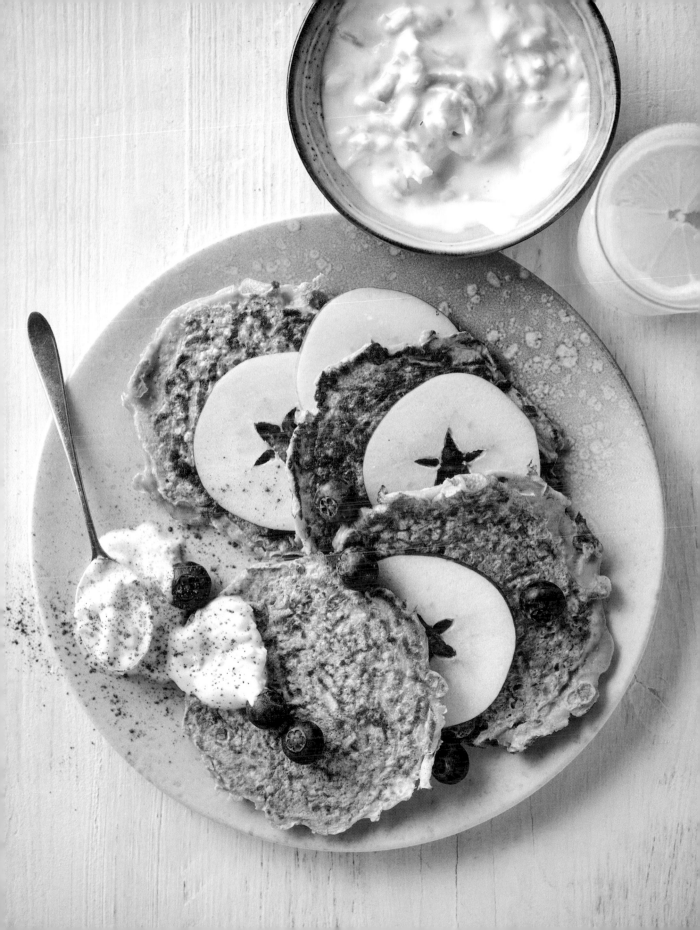

FULL *English* WRAPS

🕐 **10 MINS** | 🍲 **10 MINS** | 🔥 **220 CALS** PER SERVING

This egg wrap, filled with hearty yet low-fat classic breakfast ingredients, will revolutionize your brunch and, let's be honest … your late, post-night-out snack meals! It feels like a treat, but you'll wake up without guilt. Well … no guilt about what you ate the previous night, at least!

―――――――――――――――| *Weekly Indulgence* |―――――――――――――――

SERVES 1

1 medium egg
sea salt and freshly ground
    black pepper
low-calorie cooking spray
2 mushrooms, sliced
1 Canadian bacon medallion, diced
4 cherry tomatoes, cut into quarters
    (or 3 tbsp baked beans)
1 low-fat sausage, cooked and sliced
1 heaping tbsp grated reduced-fat
    Cheddar

Whisk the egg well and season with some salt and pepper. Set aside.

Spray a frying pan with some low-calorie cooking spray and place over a medium heat. Add the mushrooms, diced bacon and cherry tomatoes (if using) and cook for a few minutes. Just before the bacon is cooked, stir in the cooked sliced sausage and beans (if using beans rather than tomatoes). When the bacon is cooked, remove the pan from the heat and set aside.

Spray a clean, non-stick pan with some low-calorie cooking spray and place over a low heat. Pour in the beaten egg. Turn the heat up to high and cook until the top of the egg has set. Flip the egg wrap over and cook the other side. The wrap will be very thin so it should only take a couple of minutes to cook through.

Remove the wrap from the pan and put it on a plate, then spread the filling on one half. Sprinkle with the cheese, then roll or fold the wrap, cut it in half and serve.

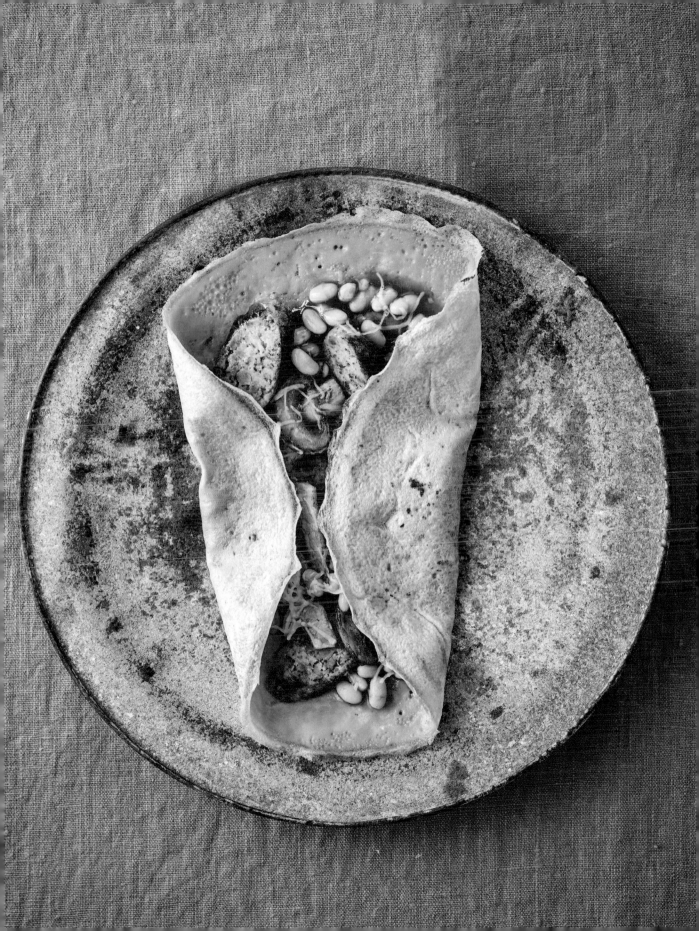

BACON, POTATO *and* SCALLION FRITTATA

🕐 **10 MINS** | 🍲 **10–15 MINS** | 🔥 **249 CALS** PER SERVING

The classic flavour combination of bacon, onion and potato works well in this easy and filling Spanish frittata. The potato makes it more substantial, the egg provides a hit of protein to curb hunger and the small amount of cheese makes it super tasty.

—————————————| *Everyday Light* |—————————————

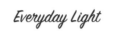

SERVES 4

7 oz medium potatoes, peeled and cut into chunks
sea salt and freshly ground black pepper
low-calorie cooking spray
1 onion, sliced
6 Canadian bacon medallions, diced
6 scallions, trimmed and chopped
8 medium eggs
1 packed tbsp chopped fresh parsley
⅓ cup reduced-fat grated Cheddar

Preheat the oven to 425°F (fan 400°F).

Cook the potato chunks in a pan of boiling salted water until soft, then drain and leave to cool.

Spray a large non-stick ovenproof frying pan with some low-calorie cooking spray and place over a medium heat. Add the sliced onion and cook for a few minutes until browned, then add the diced bacon and cook for 3 minutes until the bacon is almost cooked. Add the scallions and cook for another minute.

Meanwhile beat the eggs in a bowl and season with a little salt and pepper.

When the onions and bacon are cooked, stir in the cooked potato and the chopped parsley. Pour in the beaten eggs and cook for 2 minutes, then sprinkle the grated cheese evenly over the top and place the pan in the oven for 10–15 minutes until the egg is cooked and the cheese has melted. You can pop it under the broiler if you want the cheese a bit crispier.

Remove from the oven and serve.

Tip
You can also use skin-on new potatoes, cut into large chunks.

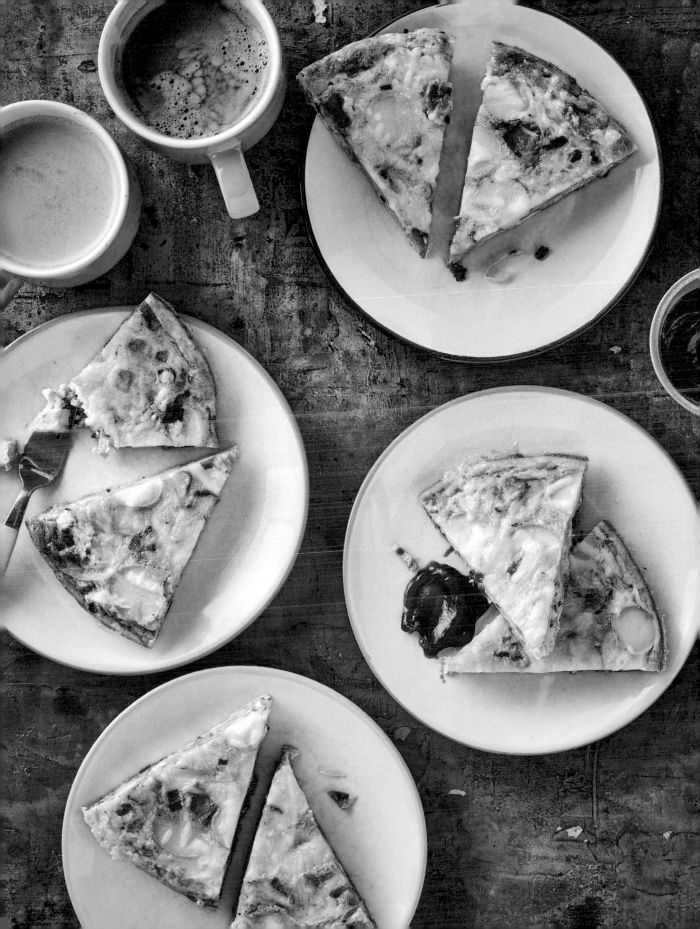

CREAMY *Mushroom* BRUSCHETTA

🕐 **5 MINS** | 🍲 **10 MINS** | 💧 **164 CALS** PER SERVING

We can't rave about these enough! One of our quickest and simplest recipes, this bruschetta is a fantastic option for a lazy breakfast, but also dinner parties and gatherings. The dish uses a deceptively small number of ingredients and is fantastically flavoursome.

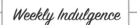

Weekly Indulgence

SERVES 2

low-calorie cooking spray
9 oz chestnut (or cremini)
    mushrooms, thickly sliced
2 garlic cloves, thinly sliced
2 gluten-free ciabattas
2 tbsp low-fat cream cheese
1 tbsp fresh basil, chopped
sea salt and freshly ground
    black pepper
1 tbsp fresh chives, snipped

Spray a frying pan with low-calorie cooking spray and place over a low–medium heat. Add the mushrooms and cook gently for a couple of minutes until they start to soften, then add the garlic and cook for another 3–4 minutes until the mushrooms are tender and the garlic is soft.

Meanwhile, cut the ciabattas in half lengthways and toast until golden. Place them on two serving plates.

Add the cream cheese to the frying pan and mix it through the mushrooms over a low heat, then add the basil and season with salt and pepper.

Top the toasted ciabatta with the creamy mushroom mix, scatter with the chives and enjoy.

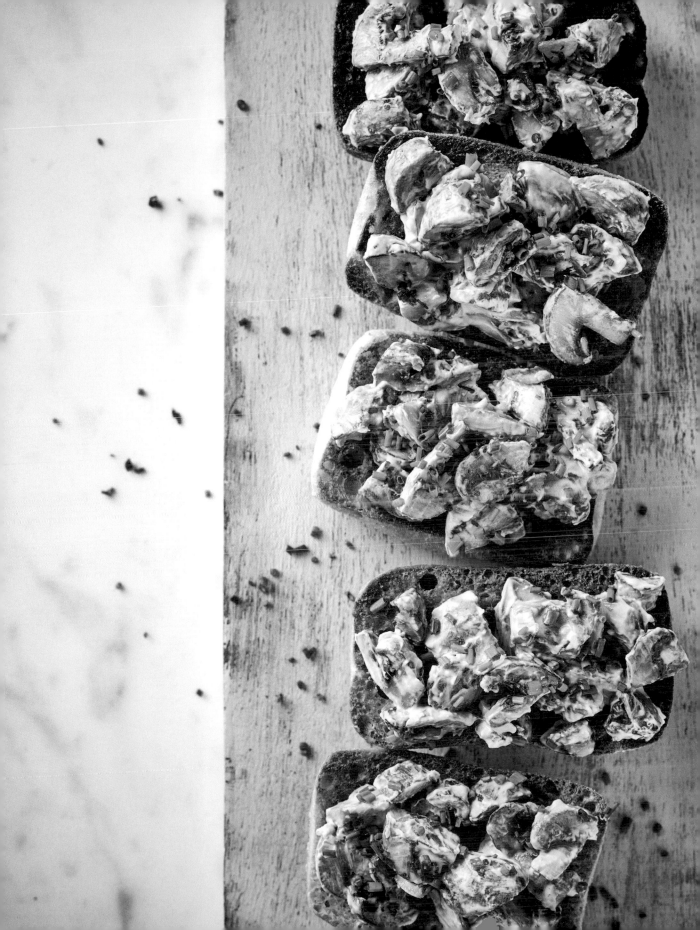

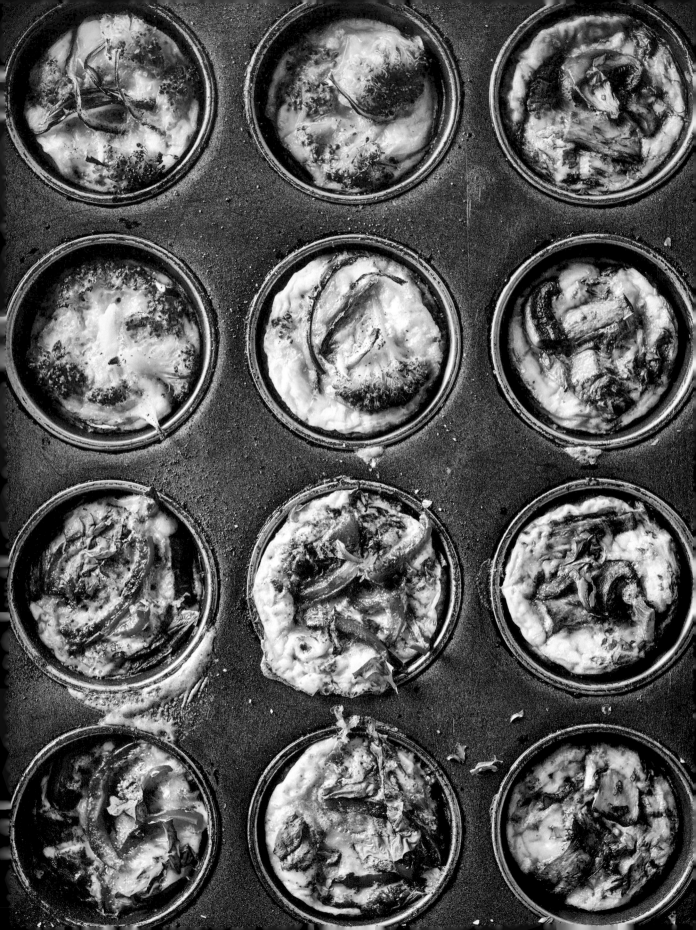

Breakfast MUFFINS

🕐 **15 MINS** | 🍲 **20 MINS** | 💧 **66 CALS** PER SERVING

Pinch of Nom staples, these muffins are perfect to make in advance for a packed lunch or a picnic, and the base mix is so versatile. We've provided three classic ideas below – each filling variation makes four muffins – but you can really add any vegetables you like.

Everyday Light

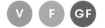

MAKES 12

FOR THE BASIC MIX
low-calorie cooking spray
12 medium eggs
sea salt and freshly ground
   black pepper

FOR GARLIC MUSHROOM MUFFINS
6 button mushrooms, sliced
2 garlic cloves, chopped
good pinch of chopped fresh parsley

**FOR SPINACH, RED PEPPER
AND PAPRIKA MUFFINS**
handful of spinach, chopped
sea salt
½ red pepper, thinly sliced
1 tsp smoked sweet paprika

**FOR BROCCOLI, RED ONION
AND BLACK PEPPER MUFFINS**
handful of cooked broccoli, chopped
½ red onion, thinly sliced
freshly ground black pepper

Preheat the oven to 350°F (fan 325°F) and spray a twelve-hole muffin tray with some low-calorie cooking spray.

Whisk the eggs well with some salt and pepper in a bowl and set aside.

To make the garlic mushroom muffins, spray a small frying pan with some low-calorie cooking spray, place over a medium heat, then add the sliced mushrooms and garlic and cook for 4 minutes until the mushrooms are soft and any moisture from the mushrooms has evaporated. Divide the mushrooms and garlic equally among four of the muffin holes.

To make the spinach, red pepper and paprika muffins, divide the chopped spinach among four of the muffin holes. Sprinkle with a little sea salt. Place the sliced red pepper on top of the spinach.

To make the broccoli, red onion and black pepper muffins, divide the cooked chopped broccoli and sliced red onion among the remaining muffin holes.

Pour the egg mix into each of the muffin cups. Top the mushroom muffins with some chopped parsley, the spinach ones with paprika and the broccoli ones with some pepper.

Bake the muffins in the oven for about 20 minutes. Serve hot or cold.

MAPLE *and* BACON
FRENCH TOAST *with* FRUIT

🕐 **5 MINS** | 🍲 **10 MINS** | 🔥 **518 CALS** PER SERVING

French toast is usually considered to be a real treat. It's hard to believe you can enjoy this while following a slimming diet. However, by using just a hint of maple syrup and some salty, lean bacon, this breakfast is delicious and indulgent, without all the calories of a traditional French toast recipe.

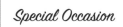

Special Occasion

SERVES 1

4 Canadian bacon medallions
2 medium eggs, beaten
1 tsp granulated sweetener
1 slice of whole-grain bread, cut into
    four triangles
low-fat cooking spray
handful of blueberries and any
    other fruit of choice
1 tbsp maple syrup

Broil or fry the bacon until it's as crispy as you like it.

Add the sweetener to the beaten eggs in a shallow bowl and stir, then soak each bread triangle in the sweetened egg mixture.

Spray a non-stick frying pan with some low-fat cooking spray and place it over a high heat. Put the bread triangles in the pan and turn the heat down to medium. Cook for 2–3 minutes until golden brown, then turn them over carefully. Cook for another 2–3 minutes. When they are golden underneath, remove them from the pan and arrange on a plate with the bacon.

Top with the blueberries and other fruit, drizzle with the maple syrup and serve.

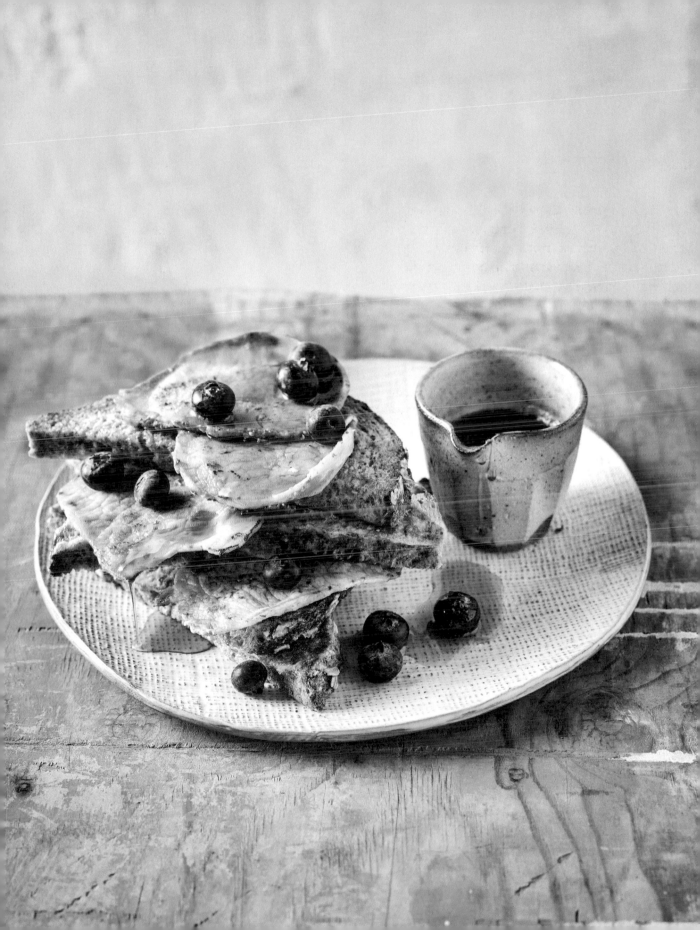

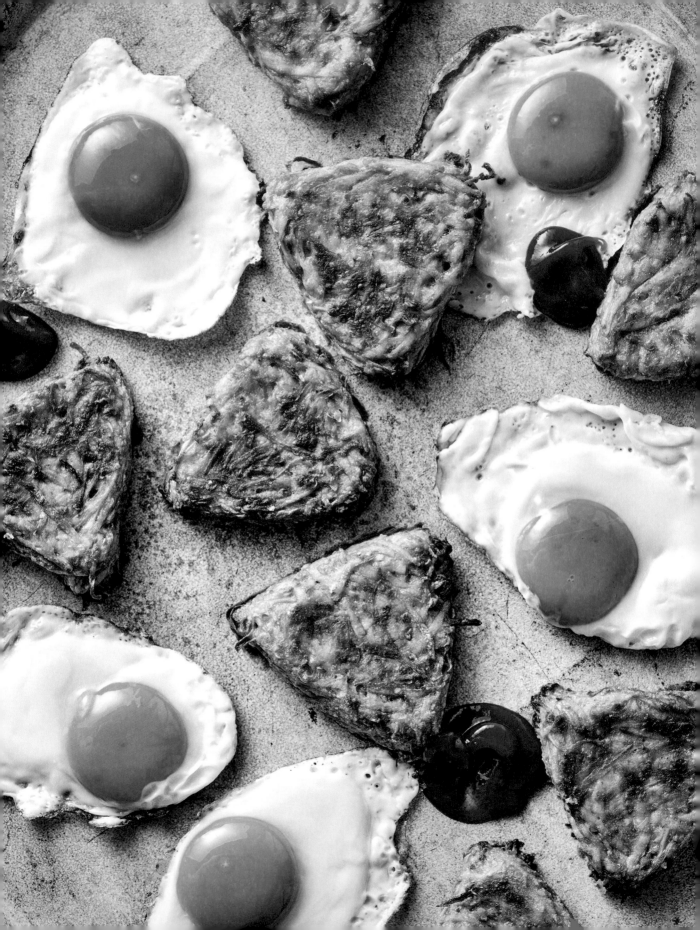

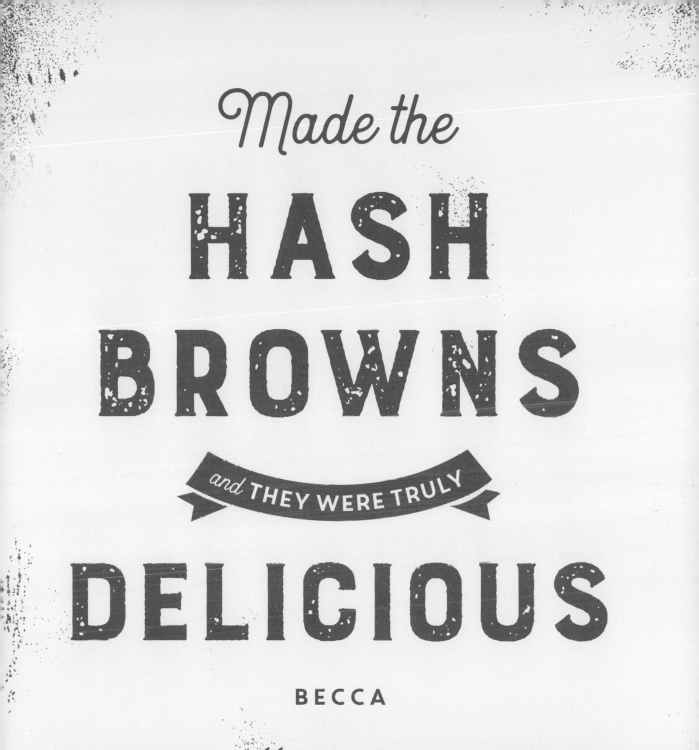

Made the
HASH
BROWNS
and THEY WERE TRULY
DELICIOUS

BECCA

"

I *loved* the **FULL ENGLISH WRAPS.** Breakfast winner!

NICOLA

We've made the **BACON, POTATO** and **SCALLION FRITTATA** for breakfast *twice* already!

EMMA

Hash BROWNS

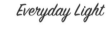 🕐 **10 MINS** | 🍲 **40 MINS** | 🔥 **77 CALS** PER SERVING

These hash browns taste just as good as the classic fry-up ones, but because you fry them in low-calorie cooking spray instead of calorific pools of oil, they are so much lighter. They are perfect for a slimming breakfast of champions! You can even make them in batches, freeze them before baking, then defrost and bake them on another day.

Everyday Light

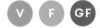 **V** **F** **GF**

SERVES 8

low-calorie cooking spray
4 large baking potatoes, peeled
1 tsp onion granules
1 medium egg
2 tsp xanthan gum
½ tsp salt
fried eggs, to serve (optional)

Preheat the oven to 375°F (fan 350°F), line a baking tray with parchment paper and spray the parchment with low-calorie cooking spray.

Coarsely grate the potatoes into a large bowl and add all the remaining ingredients. Mix together by hand – the mixture should become more starchy and sticky as you mix. Shape the potato mixture into eight flat triangle shapes (or rounds, if you prefer) and spray them with low-calorie cooking spray. (You can freeze them at this point – just pop some parchment paper between each one before freezing so you can easily separate them.)

Place on the lined baking tray and cook in the oven for 25 minutes. Spray the tops with cooking spray again, turn them over, spray the other side, and cook for another 15 minutes.

Serve the hash browns straight from the oven with fried eggs, if you like (but don't forget to count the calories).

Tip
Xanthan gum acts as an ingenious binding agent. It is a gluten-free substitute. You'll find it in "gluten-free" supermarket aisles or sections.

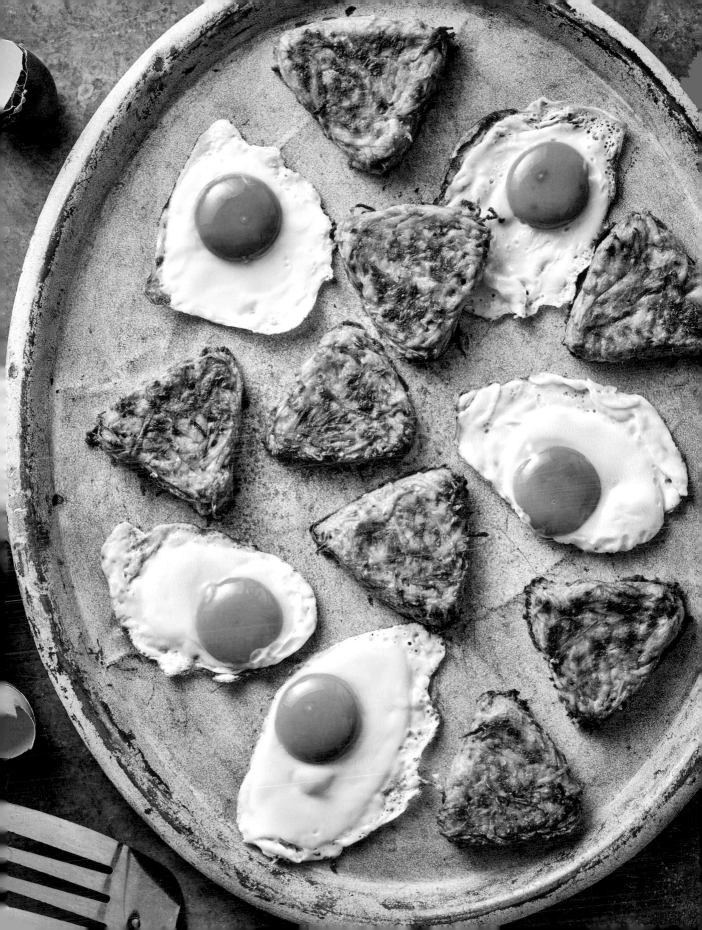

WRAPS *de* HUEVO

🕐 **10 MINS** | 🍲 **10 MINS** | 🔥 **234 CALS** PER SERVING

Once you've made these egg wraps you'll wonder how you've lived without them! An everyday staple and a great way to enjoy eggs, they are so quick, simple and easily stuffed with a variety of fillings. This version, stuffed with a tasty protein-boosting Mexican filling, is delicious cold, too, making it perfect for a packed lunch.

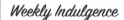

Weekly Indulgence

Ⓥ

SERVES 1

1 medium egg
sea salt and freshly ground
    black pepper
hot sauce
low-calorie cooking spray
½ small red onion, sliced
½ red pepper, sliced
pinch of garlic granules
1 cup tinned mixed beans, drained
    and rinsed
3 tbsp grated reduced-fat Cheddar
pinch of chopped fresh cilantro

Whisk the egg well and season with some salt, pepper and a dash of hot sauce. Set aside.

Spray a frying pan with some low-calorie cooking spray and place over a medium heat. Add the onion, pepper, garlic granules, mixed beans and another dash of hot sauce to the pan and cook for 4–5 minutes until the onion and pepper are just cooked. Add the cheese to the pan and stir until melted, then remove from the heat and set aside.

Spray a clean, non-stick frying pan with some low-calorie cooking spray over a high heat. When hot, pour in the beaten egg, swirling the pan so the egg covers the surface evenly and cook until the top of the wrap has set. Flip the wrap over and cook the other side. The wrap should be very thin so it should only take a couple of minutes.

Remove the wrap from the pan, then spread the filling on one half, and sprinkle a little chopped cilantro over the top. Roll or fold the wrap, cut it in half and serve.

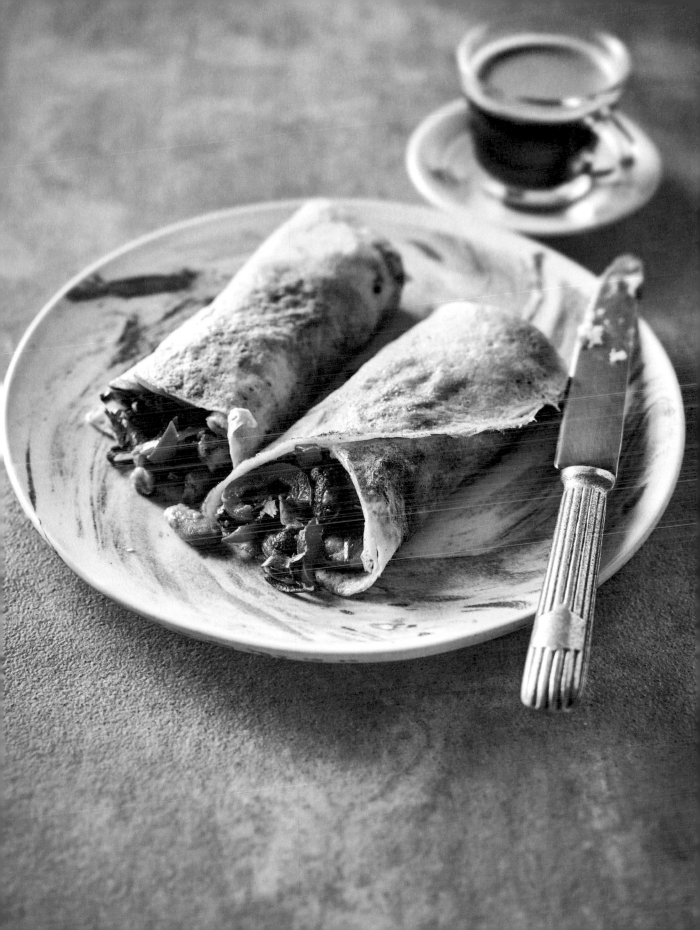

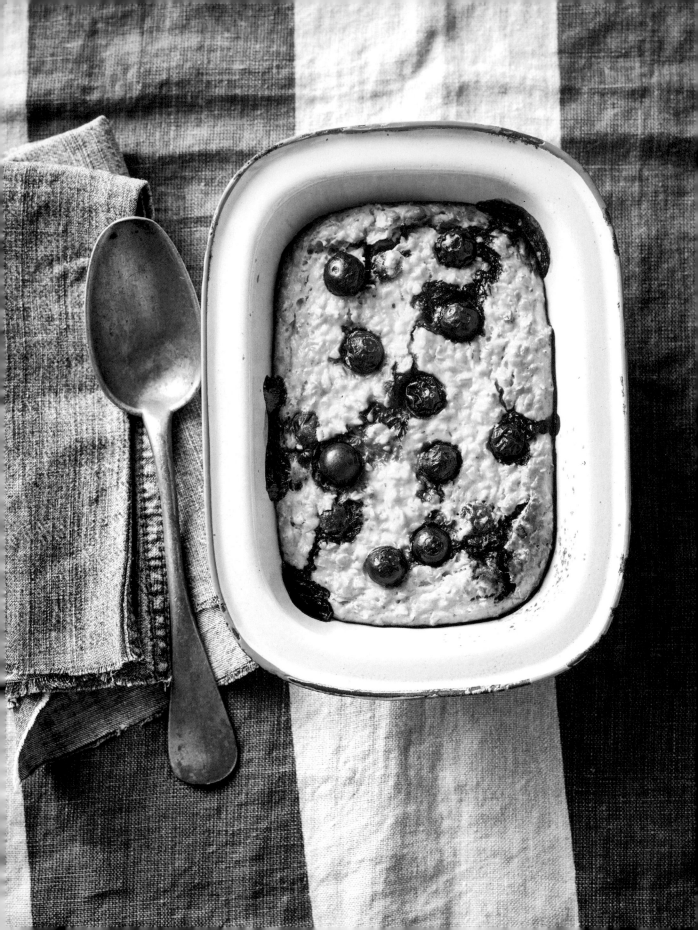

LEMON *and* BLUEBERRY BAKED OATS

🕐 **5 MINS** | 🍲 **35–40 MINS** | 🔥 **440 CALS** PER SERVING

Baked oats are a perfect warm and filling breakfast. This is one of the most popular flavour-baked oat recipes we have on the Pinch of Nom website, and it is often also used for a dessert – it feels that special.

Weekly Indulgence

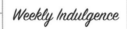

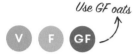

SERVES 1

½ cup rolled oats
¾ cup fat-free natural yogurt
1 tsp vanilla extract
¾ tbsp granulated sweetener
grated zest and juice of ½ lemon
2 medium eggs (or 1 medium egg if
   you prefer a slightly drier texture)
⅓ cup blueberries

Preheat the oven to 400°F (fan 375°F).

Put all of the ingredients into a bowl, keeping back a quarter of the blueberries, and stir until combined. Pour into a small ovenproof dish and place the remaining blueberries on top.

Place on a baking tray, so you don't end up with a messy oven if it rises a bit too much, and bake for 35–40 minutes.

Remove from the oven and serve warm.

Tip
You can cover and freeze the baked oats when they have cooled. Simply reheat from frozen gently in the microwave.

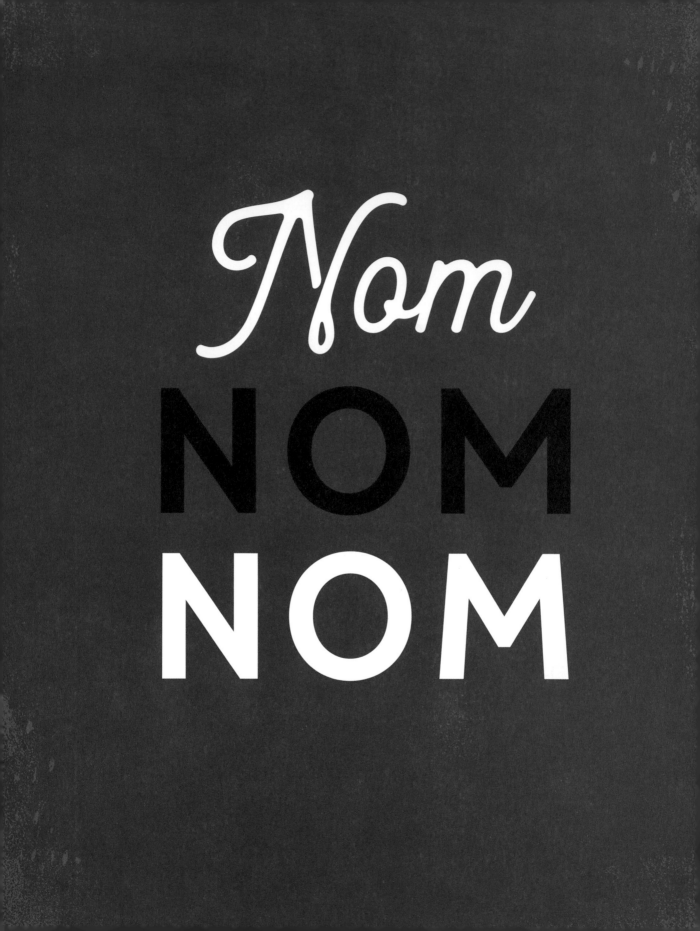

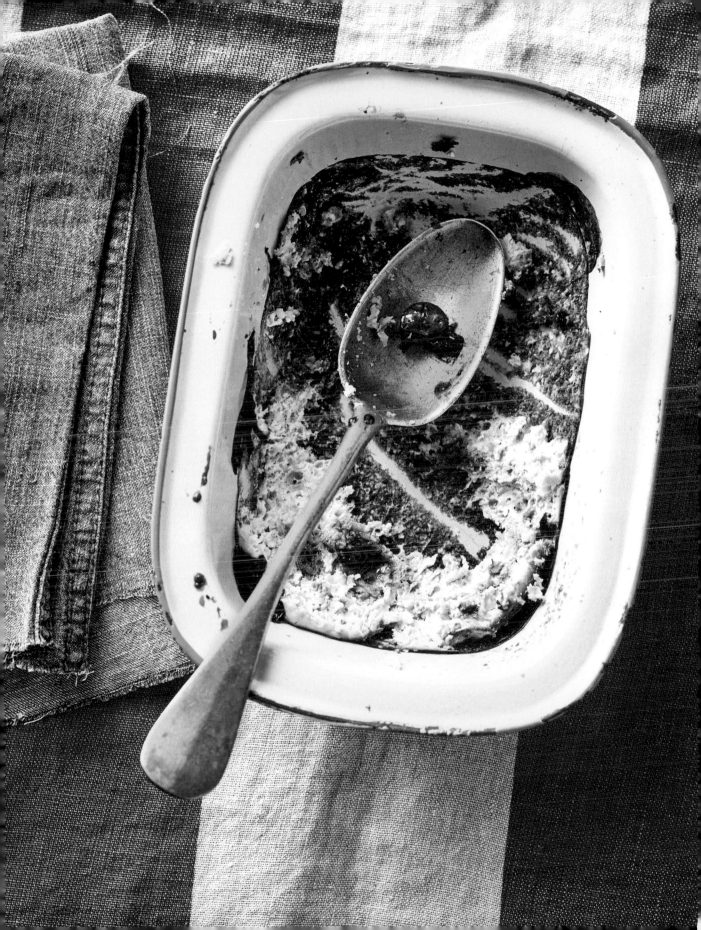

Carrot Cake
OVERNIGHT OATS

🕐 **5 MINS** | 🗑 **NO COOK** | 🔥 **318 CALS** PER SERVING

Oats have natural filling power, which means they're perfect for breakfast. This simple recipe is made the night before, so it's ready to go in the morning and great for a quick and easy start to the day. Beginning your day with a satisfying meal means you're less likely to reach for the snack drawer for something sweet before lunch. You can also make this gluten-free by using a gluten-free cereal, such as Oatabix.

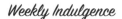

Weekly Indulgence

V

SERVES 1

½ cup rolled oats or 2 Weetabix, crushed
1 (6-oz) cup vanilla-flavoured fat-free yogurt (or fat-free natural yogurt, ½ tsp vanilla extract and ½–1 tsp granulated sweetener)
1 small carrot, grated
¼ tsp mixed spice (or pumpkin pie spice)
pinch of ground ginger
pinch of ground cinnamon

Put the oats or Weetabix in the bottom of a canning jar or a jar with a lid. Spoon the yogurt and three-quarters of the carrot on top and add the spices. Stir well until completely combined, then cover and chill in the fridge overnight.

The next morning, stir, top with the reserved grated carrot and enjoy.

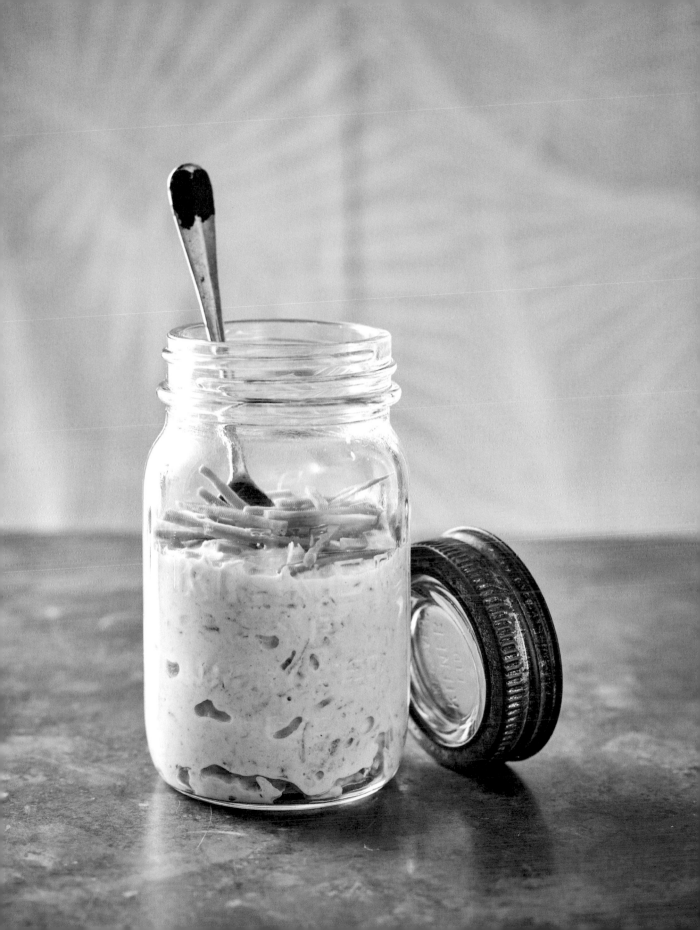

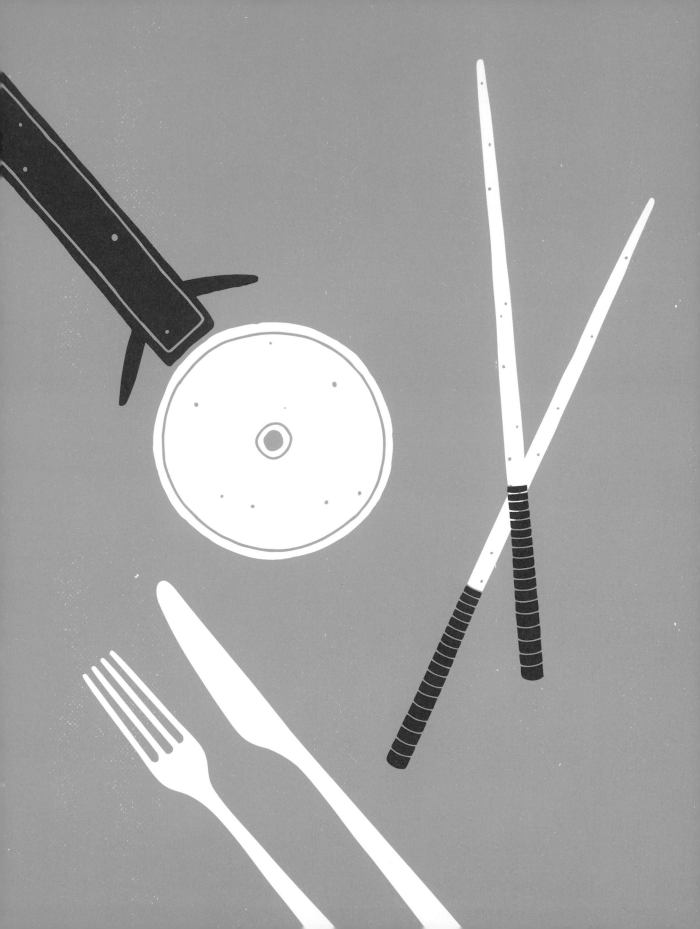

CHAPTER 2

FAKEAWAYS

Tandoori
CHICKEN KEBAB

🕐 **5 MINS** (PLUS MARINATING TIME) | 🍲 **30 MINS** | 💧 **236 CALS** PER SERVING

Tandoori chicken is traditionally prepared by roasting chicken, marinated in yogurt and spices, in a tandoor clay oven. However, we suggest using the grill to the same effect in this recipe. You can also use the oven on a rainy day without any bother. The marinade makes the chicken really tender and tasty.

— | *Everyday Light* | —

Use GF soy sauce

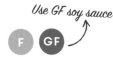

SERVES 4

1⅓ cups fat-free Greek-style yogurt plus extra to serve (optional)
4 tbsp tandoori spice mix
1 garlic clove, finely grated
1 tbsp finely grated fresh ginger
juice of ½ lemon
1 tsp dark soy sauce
½ tsp salt
1–2 drops of red food colouring (optional)
1 lb 5 oz chicken thigh fillets (skin and visible fat removed), cut into large chunks
green salad, to serve

Put all of the ingredients (except the chicken) in a bowl and stir thoroughly. Add the chicken to the yogurt marinade, cover and chill in the fridge for 2–4 hours.

Preheat the oven to 400°F (fan 375°F) or fire up the grill.

Remove the chicken from the fridge. Thread the chicken onto skewers. (You can use metal or bamboo skewers, but soak bamboo skewers in water first to prevent them from burning.)

Place the skewers on the grill and cook for 30–35 minutes until the chicken has cooked through. If you're cooking them in the oven, skewer the meat as above, place the skewers on a baking tray and cook in the oven for 35–40 minutes until cooked through.

Serve the kebabs with green salad and more yogurt, if desired (but don't forget to count the calories).

Tip
You can freeze the marinated skewers on trays before cooking. Simply defrost and cook as per the recipe.

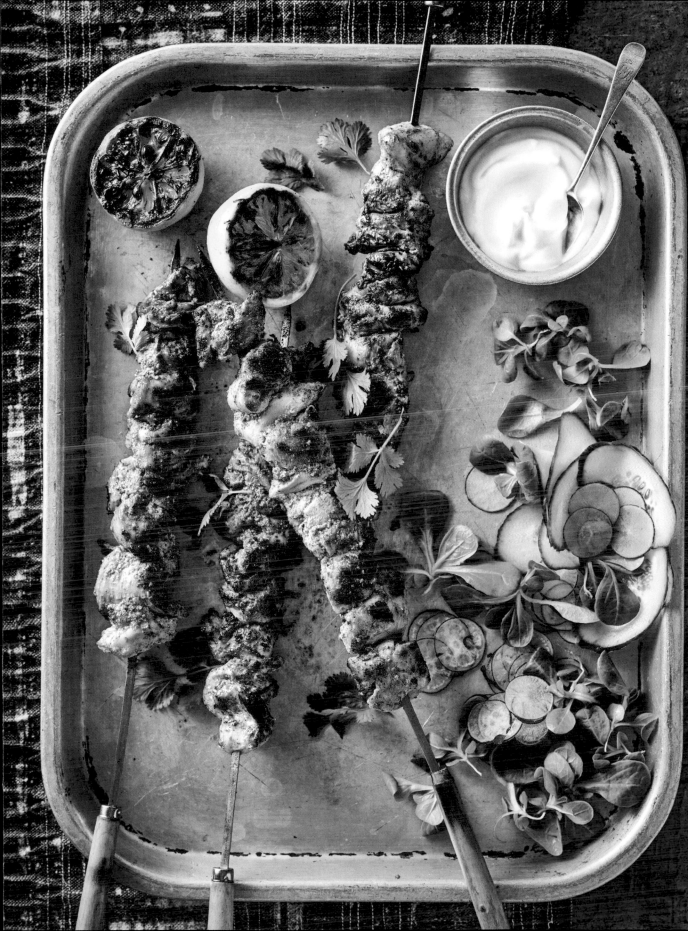

Chicken BALTI

🕐 **15 MINS** (PLUS MARINATING TIME) | 🍲 **30 MINS** | 💧 **373 CALS** PER SERVING

Using fresh ingredients for this flavoursome balti means you get that authentic takeaway flavour, while keeping a handle on the calories. Scale up the ingredients for the balti paste and portion it off for freezing, so you have an easy curry base on hand for whenever the Indian takeaway craving pops up!

— *Everyday Light* —

Use GF stock cubes

SERVES 4

4 chicken breasts (skin and visible fat removed), diced
1 cinnamon stick or 1 tsp ground cinnamon
½ tsp dried chile flakes
½ cup plus 2 tbsp chicken stock (½ chicken stock cube, dissolved in ½ cup plus 2 tbsp boiling water)
1 (14 oz) tin chopped tomatoes
1 chicken stock cube
1 red pepper, deseeded and cut into strips
1 yellow pepper, deseeded and cut into strips
1 orange pepper, deseeded and cut into strips
sea salt (optional)
1 tsp garam masala

FOR THE BALTI PASTE
low-calorie cooking spray
2 large onions, roughly chopped
½ in piece of fresh ginger, peeled and chopped
2 garlic cloves, roughly chopped
1 tsp ground turmeric
½ tsp dried chile flakes
2 tbsp smoked sweet paprika
2 tsp ground cumin
2 tsp ground coriander
1 tsp ground cinnamon
1 tsp salt
½ tsp freshly ground black pepper
3 tbsp tomato paste

TO SERVE (OPTIONAL)
handful of fresh cilantro leaves, roughly chopped
Onion Bhajis (see page 204)
cooked rice

Start by making the balti paste. Spray a frying pan with low-calorie cooking spray and place over a medium heat. Add the onions, ginger and garlic to the pan and fry for 3–4 minutes until the onion is golden brown.

Put the contents of the pan and the rest of the paste ingredients in a food processor or blender and blitz until it forms a paste. Transfer to a bowl, allow to cool and put in the fridge, or – if you're making ahead – freeze it in an ice-cube tray.

Place the chicken in a freezer bag or bowl. Add 4 tablespoons of the paste, mix well and place in the fridge to marinate for an hour or so.

Spray a large frying pan with low-calorie cooking spray and place over a medium heat. Add the cinnamon and chile flakes and cook for 2 minutes, then spray the pan with more cooking spray, add 4 tablespoons of the balti paste and cook for another 2 minutes. Add the stock, tinned tomatoes and stock cube, stir well and bring to the boil, then turn the heat down to medium, add the marinated chicken and pepper strips and cook for 15 minutes.

Taste the curry and add more salt if you like, and check that the chicken is cooked through. Stir in the garam masala, cook for another 3 minutes and serve garnished with the cilantro, if using.

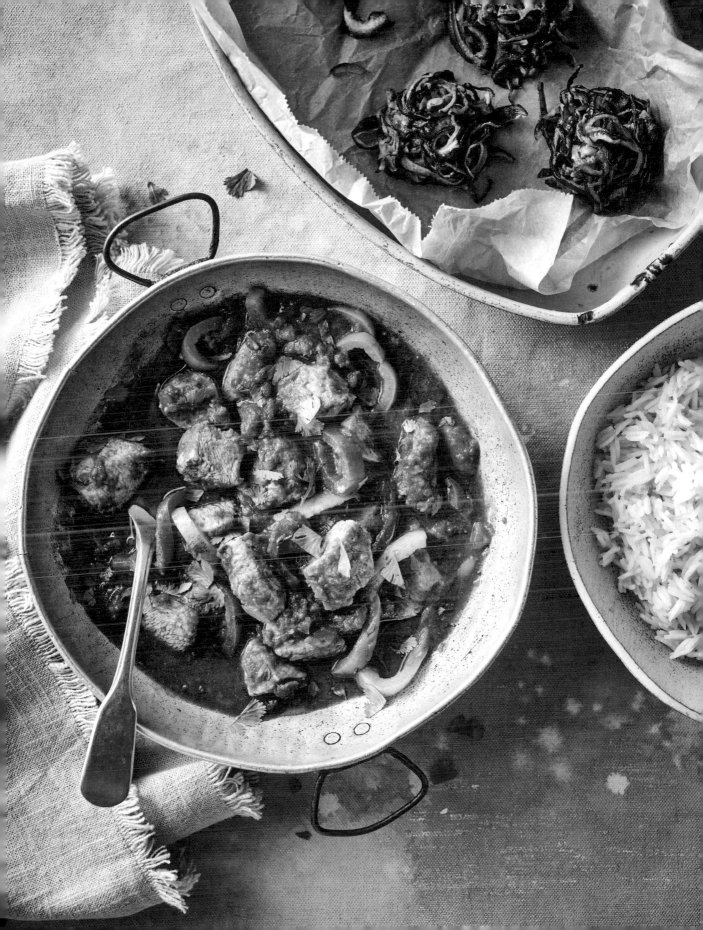

CHICKEN *and* MUSHROOM STIR FRY

🕐 **10 MINS** | 🍲 **20 MINS** | 🔥 **274 CALS** PER SERVING

One of the most common requests we receive is for quick and simple fakeaway recipes. This chicken and mushroom Chinese-style fakeaway is a Pinch of Nom classic. With fresh ingredients and authentic flavours of soy and oyster sauce, you'll never need to call for a takeaway again.

── *Everyday Light* ──

F

SERVES 2

low-calorie cooking spray
1 onion, sliced
2 chicken breasts (skin and visible fat removed), diced
1 red pepper, deseeded and sliced
1 green pepper, deseeded and sliced
handful of broccoli florets
1 garlic clove, crushed
½ tsp finely chopped fresh ginger
6 scallions, trimmed and chopped
handful of baby corn, roughly chopped
7 oz button mushrooms, sliced
4 tbsp soy sauce
2 tbsp oyster sauce
2 tbsp rice vinegar (or white wine vinegar with a little sweetener added)
¼ tsp freshly ground black pepper
1 cup beef stock (1 beef stock cube dissolved in 1 cup boiling water)
cooked rice or noodles, to serve

Spray a wok or large frying pan with low-calorie cooking spray and place it over a medium heat.

Add the onion, chicken, peppers, broccoli, garlic and ginger and stir-fry for 3 minutes until the onions and peppers start to soften. Add the scallions, baby corn and mushrooms and stir-fry for 3 minutes until they start to colour slightly, then add the soy sauce, oyster sauce, rice vinegar and black pepper.

Pour in the stock, stir well and turn the heat up to high. Simmer until the sauce reduces and thickens slightly. Check the chicken is cooked through and serve with rice or noodles.

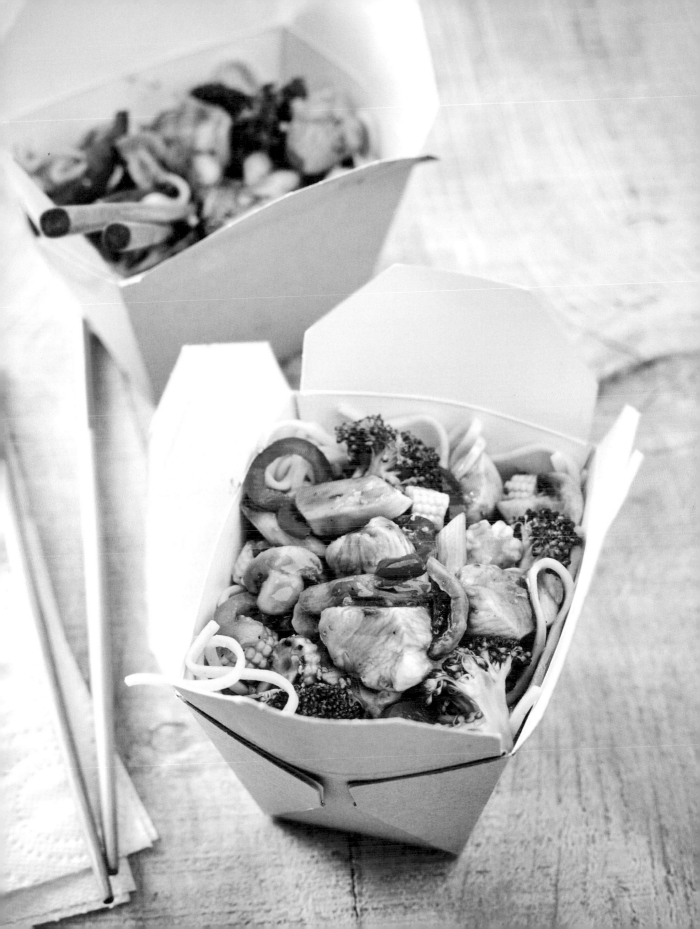

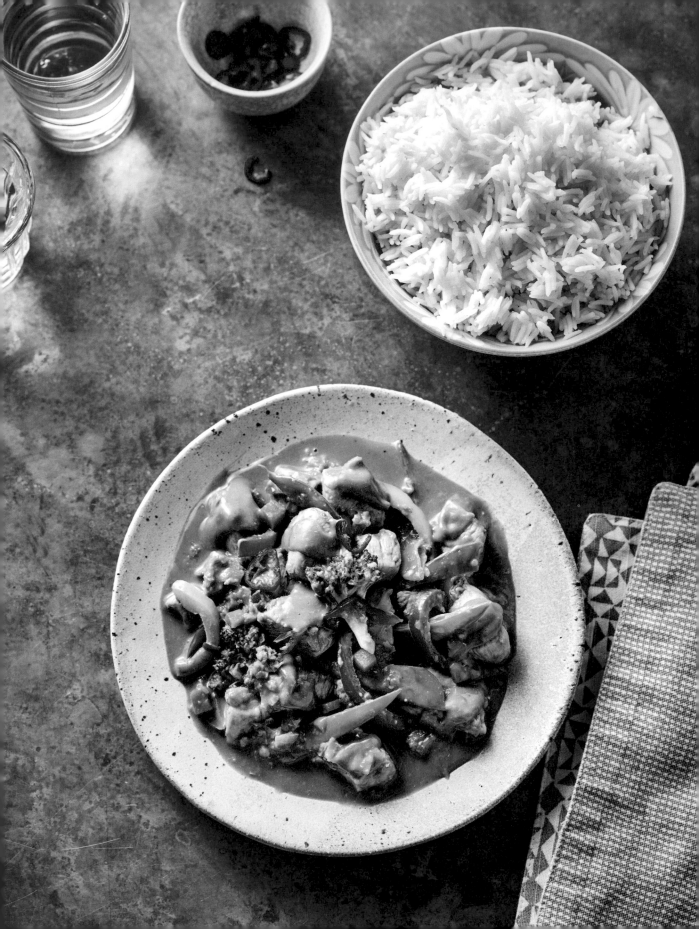

Chicken SATAY

🕐 **20 MINS** | 🍲 **30 MINS** | 🔥 **293 CALS** PER SERVING

This ingredient-heavy recipe may seem a little daunting, but we promise it's worth that little bit of extra effort. The ingredients are mostly all store-cupboard ingredients that you probably already have lurking in the kitchen. The rich peanut sauce cleverly uses dehydrated peanut powder, which instantly cuts out the fats of normal peanut butter, while packing the same big flavour.

Weekly Indulgence

Use GF soy sauce

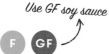

SERVES 6

½ onion, sliced
4 chicken breasts (skin and visible fat removed), diced
2 medium carrots, finely chopped
handful of broccoli florets
3½ oz snow peas
1 red pepper, deseeded and sliced
1 yellow pepper, deseeded and sliced
4 scallions, trimmed and chopped
1 tbsp light soy sauce
cooked rice, to serve

FOR THE SAUCE
low-calorie cooking spray
½ onion, finely chopped
3 garlic cloves, finely chopped
thumb-sized piece of fresh ginger, peeled and finely chopped
1 red chile, chopped (leave the seeds in if you like it hotter)
¼ tsp ground cumin
½ tsp ground coriander
1 tbsp ground turmeric
3 tbsp light soy sauce
1 tbsp fish sauce or Worcestershire sauce
3 tbsp granulated sweetener
2½ cups unsweetened coconut water
4 tbsp reduced-fat peanut butter powder
generous pinch of sea salt
2 tbsp cornstarch

To make the sauce, spray a frying pan with low-calorie cooking spray, place over a medium heat, add the the onion, garlic, ginger and chile and fry for 4–5 minutes until the onion has softened. Add the dry spices and stir for 1 minute, then add all the other sauce ingredients apart from the cornstarch. Simmer over a medium heat for 10 minutes, then blitz with a stick blender (or transfer to a blender or food processor, blitz until smooth and return the sauce to the pan).

Turn the heat up to high. Mix the cornstarch with a little water, stir it into the simmering sauce until it thickens, then remove from the heat and set aside.

To make the satay chicken, spray a wok with low-calorie cooking spray, place over a high heat, add the onion and chicken and fry for 5 minutes until the onion softens. Add the vegetables and the soy sauce and stir-fry for a few minutes, then add the sauce.

Turn down the heat and simmer for 10 minutes, making sure the chicken is cooked through. Serve with rice.

Philly CHEESESTEAK

🕐 **5 MINS** | 🍲 **10 MINS** | 🔥 **375 CALS** PER SERVING

A good Philly cheesesteak is a favourite we can't quite forget, so we decided to re-create this classic dish. Using a gluten-free ciabatta and being savvy with the base sauce ingredients can avoid an overload of calories. Have no fear though, it'll still give you a tasty, indulgent Philly cheesesteak that satisfies every craving!

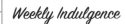

Weekly Indulgence

SERVES 2

5¼ oz steak (all visible fat removed),
   cut into super-thin slices
sea salt and freshly ground
   black pepper
low-calorie cooking spray
4 mushrooms, sliced
½ onion, sliced
½ pepper (green, red or yellow),
   deseeded and sliced
5 tbsp light spreadable cheese
2 gluten-free ciabatta rolls,
   split lengthways

Season the steak well with salt and pepper and set it aside for 1 minute.

Spray a non-stick frying pan with some low-calorie cooking spray, place over a high heat, add the steak slices and cook for 3–4 minutes, or until cooked through. Remove them from the pan and transfer to a bowl.

Spray the pan with a little more low-calorie cooking spray, then add the mushrooms, onion and pepper and cook for 3–4 minutes until they soften. Remove from the heat.

Stir the spreadable cheese into the steak and mix well, then add the steak to the pan with the veg and stir.

Fill the two ciabatta rolls with equal quantities of the steak mix, replace the top of the roll, and serve.

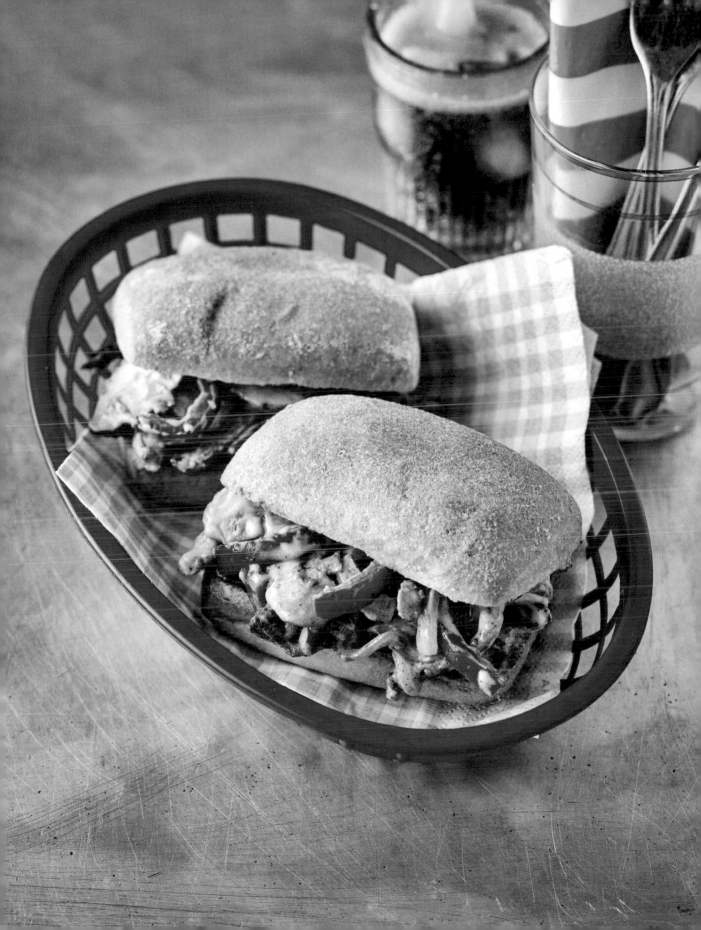

Super Simple CHICKEN CURRY

🕐 **5 MINS** | 🗑 **30 MINS** | 🔥 **181 CALS** PER SERVING

Occasionally, the craving for a good Indian dish is overwhelming. We would all love to have the opportunity to create curry pastes and spice mixes from scratch. At times though, we just need a quick, easy, go-to curry recipe that can be created in minutes. This is one such recipe. Wonderfully tasty, but so quick to put together, it'll become a regular evening meal in no time.

Everyday Light

SERVES 4

low-calorie cooking spray
1 large onion, sliced
1 lb chicken breast (skin and
    visible fat removed), diced
3 garlic cloves, crushed
1⅔ cups water
3 tbsp curry powder
2 tsp ground turmeric
1 tbsp tomato paste
sea salt and freshly ground
    black pepper

TO SERVE (OPTIONAL)
Samosas (see page 224)
cooked rice

Spray a large frying pan with low-calorie cooking spray and place over a medium heat. Add the onion and cook for 2 minutes until softened slightly, then add the diced chicken to the pan and cook for 5 minutes until browned.

Add the garlic to the pan and cook for 1 minute, then add all the other ingredients. The water should just about cover the chicken – you may need a little more or less depending on the size of your pan.

Leave to simmer gently for 20 minutes.

Turn the heat up and boil the curry for another 5 minutes, stirring frequently to ensure it doesn't catch on the bottom of the pan – this will reduce and thicken the sauce slightly.

Serve the curry with your choice of accompaniment.

Tip
This curry recipe works well with lean diced lamb (all visible fat removed), too.

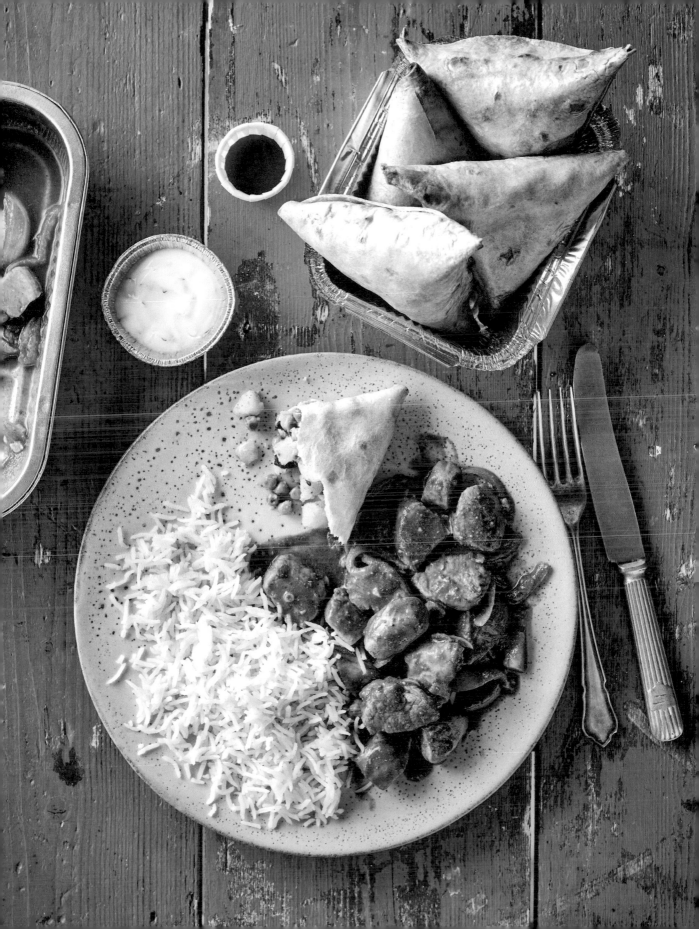

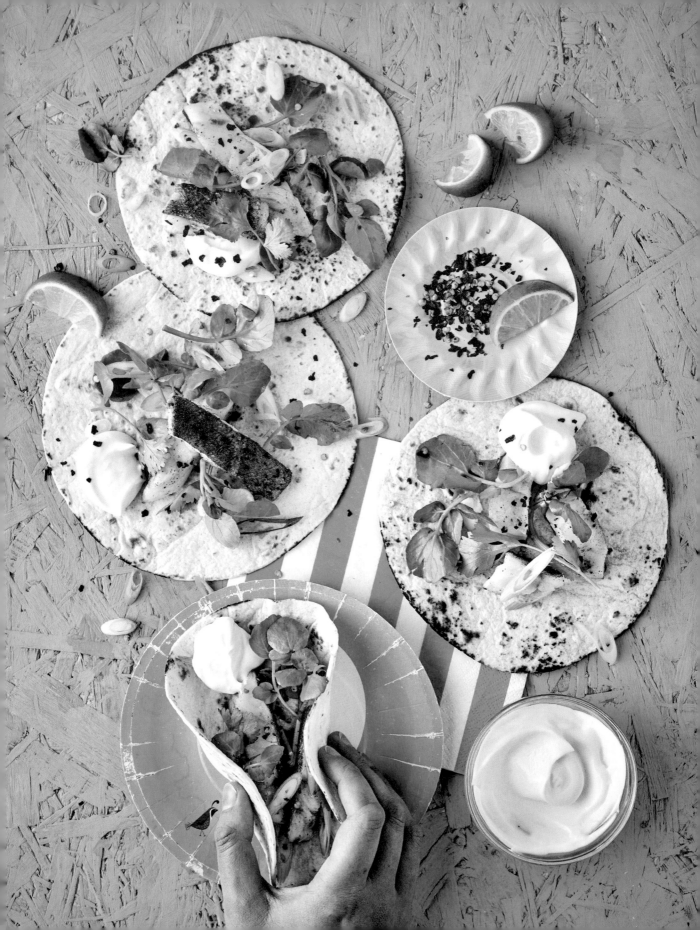

SOFT *Fish* TACOS

🕐 **5 MINS** | 🍲 **10 MINS** | 🔥 **190 CALS** PER SERVING

A beautifully light dish, this recipe treats white fish with the delicacy it deserves, while delivering wonderfully fresh flavours with the chile and scallion. These tacos are perfect for all occasions – ideal for kids who'll love stacking their own, and adults for a quick evening meal.

--- *Everyday Light* ---

Use GF wraps

SERVES 2

2 small fillets of white fish (about 10 oz), preferably skin on, cut into strips about 1¼ in wide
¼ tsp mild chile powder
¼ tsp garlic granules
¼ tsp ground coriander
low-calorie cooking spray
pinch of salt
small handful of watercress or arugula
a few sprigs of fresh cilantro
1 scallion, trimmed and chopped
2 low-calorie tortilla wraps, halved (or 4 small ones)
wedge of lime
4 tsp fat-free Greek-style yogurt, plus extra to serve (optional)
pinch of dried chile flakes

Place the strips of fish – you should have about eight – skin side up on a board and sprinkle with the chile powder, garlic granules and ground coriander.

Spray a frying pan with low-calorie cooking spray and place over a high heat. Add the fish to the pan, skin side down, and cook for 4 minutes – do not be tempted to flip the fillets or move them, you want the skin to be crisp!

Spray the fillets with low-calorie cooking spray, then flip the fish over. Sprinkle over the salt and cook for 2 minutes.

Meanwhile, place your choice of leaves, the fresh cilantro and some chopped scallion onto each half wrap.

When the fish is cooked, place a couple of strips onto each prepared wrap. Squeeze over a little lime juice, dollop a blob of fat-free yogurt and give each taco a little pinch of chile flakes, then serve.

Tip
This works best with fish fillets that have the skin on, as it goes really crisp and adds an amazing texture.

VEGETABLE BIRYANI

🕐 **15 MINS** | 🍲 **10 MINS** | 🔥 **302 CALS** PER SERVING

Bursting with spices and flavours, a biryani is a baked rice dish that packs a real punch. Made with loads of beautiful vegetables, this is a healthy and satisfying meal with masses of flavour. The egg provides both the protein and an extra layer of texture to the dish.

Everyday Light

Use a GF stock cube

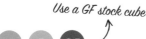

SERVES 4

low-calorie cooking spray
1 cup plus 2 tbsp basmati rice
2 garlic cloves, finely chopped
1 tbsp medium curry powder
2⅔ cups vegetable stock (1 vegetable stock cube dissolved in 2⅔ cups boiling water)
1 orange pepper, deseeded and diced
6 scallions, trimmed and chopped
¾ cup sugar snap peas, each sliced into 3 pieces
1⅓ cups broccoli cut into small florets
1⅓ cups cauliflower cut into small florets
⅓ cup frozen peas
⅓ cup sweet corn kernels (tinned and drained, or frozen)
handful of chopped fresh cilantro
3 medium eggs
sea salt and freshly ground black pepper
juice of ½ lemon

Spray a saucepan with some low-calorie cooking spray and place over a medium heat. Add the rice, garlic and curry powder and fry for 1–2 minutes, stirring, then add the stock. Stir well, turn the heat down to low, cover and simmer for 10–15 minutes, according to the instructions on the packet of rice. It's ready when the rice is cooked and all the stock has been absorbed.

While the rice is cooking, spray a frying pan or wok with some more low-calorie cooking spray, place over a medium heat, and add all the veg. Fry for about 10 minutes, stirring continuously – don't overcook the veg as you want them to remain crunchy.

When the rice is cooked, remove the lid, add the cooked veg and stir in most of the cilantro. Replace the lid to keep it hot.

Whisk the eggs in a bowl and add some salt and pepper.

Spray a clean pan with some low-calorie cooking spray and place over a medium heat. Pour in the egg and cook on one side for 1–2 minutes, then flip it over to make an omelette and remove it from the pan.

Stir the lemon juice through the rice, then cut the omelette into slices and arrange it on top. Sprinkle with the remaining cilantro and serve.

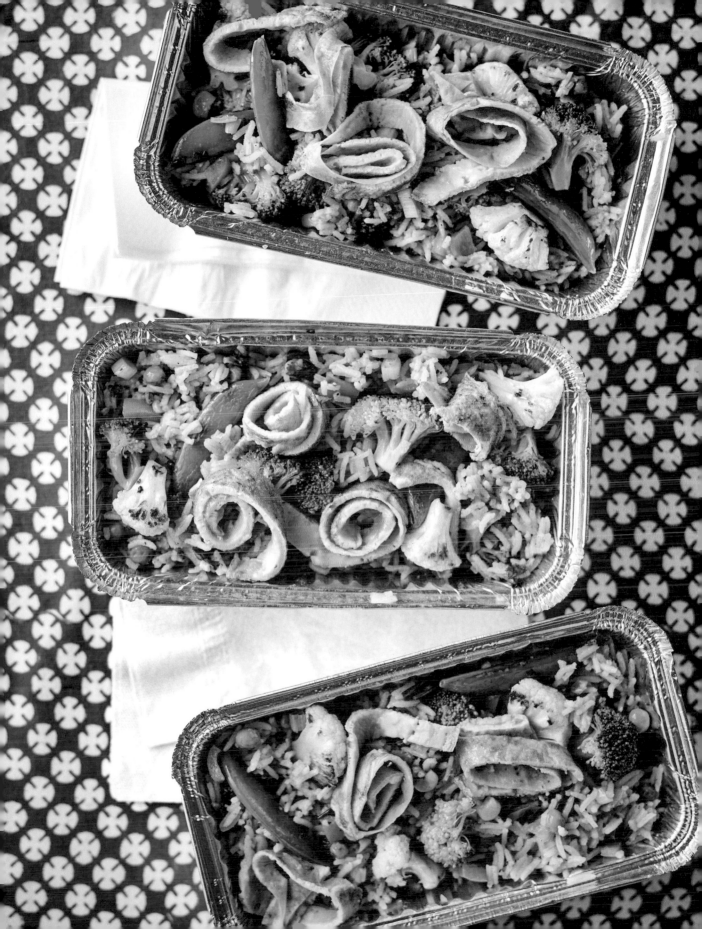

BBQ CHICKEN
DRUMSTICKS *and* THIGHS

🕐 **25 MINS** | 🍲 **30 MINS** | 🔥 **218 CALS** PER SERVING

There's no reason why you shouldn't enjoy a good barbecue when following a healthier diet. Preparation, as ever, is key. You can make the rich barbecue sauce in advance, and coat the chicken in the sauce and seasoning in advance, too, ready for cooking. Just cook the coated chicken when you're ready – in the oven if it's not barbecue weather – and smother it with the remaining sauce to serve.

Everyday Light

SERVES 4

4 chicken drumsticks (skin and
  visible fat removed)
4 bone-in chicken thighs (skin and
  visible fat removed)
1 tbsp BBQ seasoning
green salad, to serve

FOR THE BBQ SAUCE
low-calorie cooking spray
½ onion, diced
2 garlic cloves, chopped
1 tbsp tomato paste
1 (14 oz) tin chopped tomatoes
juice of ½ lemon
1 tbsp BBQ seasoning
1 tbsp balsamic vinegar
2 tbsp Worcestershire sauce
  (or use a suitable GF substitute)
2 tbsp white wine vinegar
1 tbsp buffalo wings hot sauce
1 tsp English mustard powder
1 tsp granulated sweetener

To make the BBQ sauce, spray a frying pan with low-calorie cooking spray, place over a medium heat, add the onion and garlic and cook for 4–5 minutes until the onions have softened. Add the tomato paste and tinned tomatoes and cook for 5 minutes over a high heat, stirring frequently, then add the rest of the ingredients, turn down the heat and simmer for 20 minutes until the sauce has thickened nicely. If the sauce seems a bit too thick just add a little water and stir well.

You can use the BBQ sauce as it is, or if you prefer a smoother sauce, just blitz it in a food processor or with a stick blender until you get the desired consistency. (You can store in a sterilized airtight container in the fridge for up to 3 days until ready to use or freeze for serving on another day.)

Place the chicken portions in an ovenproof dish. Sprinkle with the BBQ seasoning and coat with a few tablespoons of the BBQ sauce. (You can do this the day before you wish to serve, if you like, or cover and freeze for cooking on another day.)

Preheat the oven to 400°F (fan 375°F) or fire up the grill.

Cook the chicken in the oven or on the grill for 30 minutes, or until cooked through (if you are cooking the chicken in the oven it may be ready after 20 minutes). Check that the juices run clear when you insert a knife into the thickest part of the thighs. Remove from the oven and serve with the remaining sauce, hot or cold.

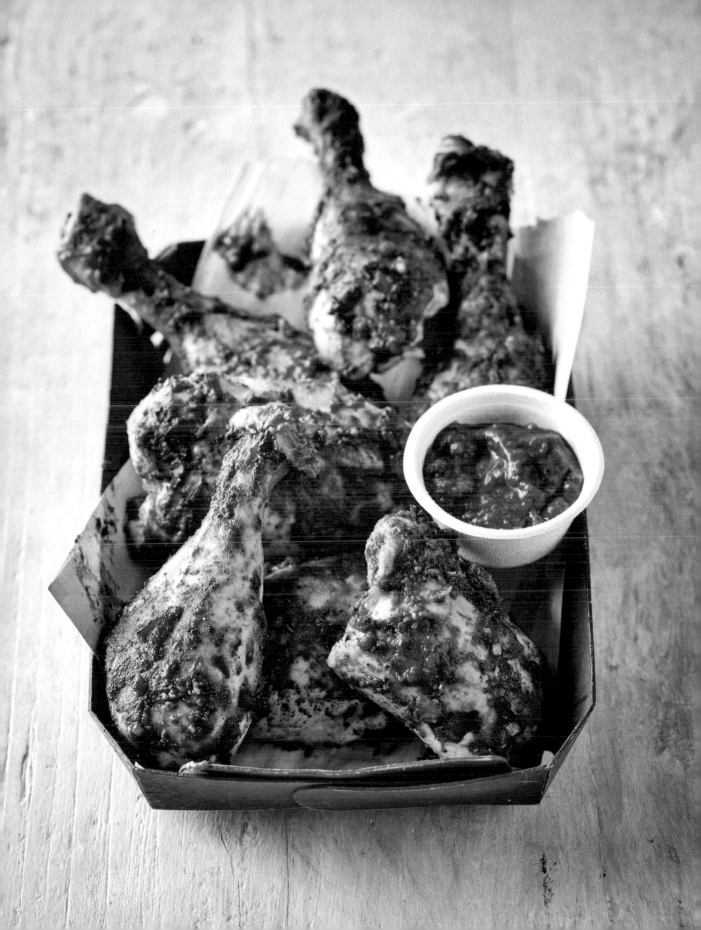

Doner KEBAB

🕐 **10 MINS** | 🍲 **VARIABLE** (SEE BELOW) | 🔥 **170 CALS** PER SERVING

This recipe combines some clever seasoning with simple minced beef to create a tasty, guilt-free fakeaway. Slow-cooking the ingredients retains the flavour and means you can throw the ingredients in before work and come home to a takeaway already delivered. You can even freeze it once cooked (provided the minced beef hasn't already been frozen).

Everyday Light

F

SERVES 4

low-calorie cooking spray
   (if cooking in the oven)
1 lb 2 oz 5%-fat ground beef
½ tsp onion granules
1 tsp ground cumin
½ tsp garlic granules
¼ tsp smoked sweet paprika
½ tsp ground coriander
1 tsp dried oregano
1 tsp dried mixed herbs
¼ tsp cayenne pepper
1 tsp sea salt
pinch of freshly ground black pepper

TO SERVE (OPTIONAL)
whole-wheat pita bread
green salad
low-fat natural yogurt mixed with
   mint sauce

OVEN METHOD
🍲 **1 HOUR 45 MINS**

Preheat the oven to 350°F (fan 325°F). Spray a 9 × 5 × 3-in non-stick loaf tin with a little low-calorie cooking spray.

Place the remaining ingredients in a blender or food processor and blitz until fairly smooth. Remove from the blender and place the mixture into the tin, pressing it down into the corners firmly.

Cover the tin with foil and cook for 1 hour 20 minutes, then remove the foil and continue cooking for another 10 minutes.

Leave to rest for 10–15 minutes, then remove from the tin, slice thinly and serve with the bread, salad and yogurt.

ELECTRIC PRESSURE COOKER METHOD
🍲 **45 MINS**

Put all of the ingredients in a blender or food processor and blitz until fairly smooth.

Form the meat into a meatloaf shape. Wrap tightly in foil, making sure there are no gaps. Place the trivet in the pressure cooker and place the wrapped meat on top.

Add 1 cup water to the pot and set the pressure cooker to Manual/Stew for 30 minutes. Allow the pressure to release naturally (Natural Pressure Release/NPR). Remove from the cooker, then leave to rest for 10–15 minutes. Remove from the foil, slice thinly and serve with the bread, salad and yogurt.

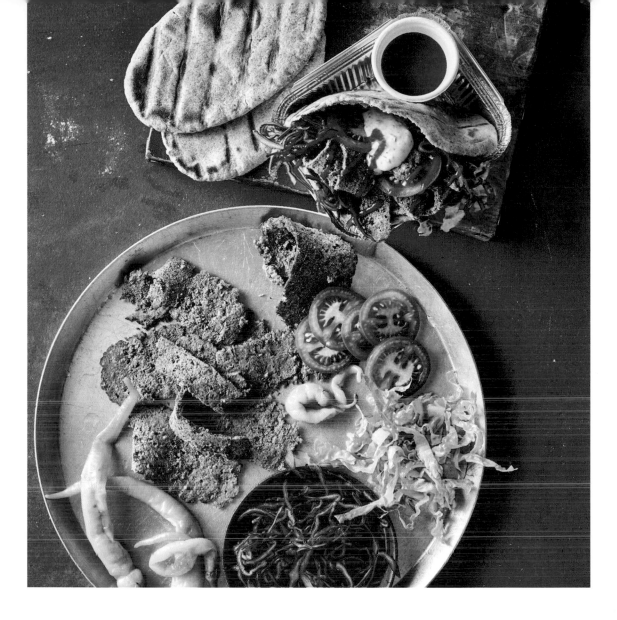

SLOW COOKER METHOD
🥘 4½ HOURS

Put all of the ingredients in a blender or food processor and blitz until fairly smooth. Remove from the blender or food processor and form the meat into a meatloaf shape. Wrap it tightly in foil, making sure there are no gaps. Place three small balls of foil in the bottom of the slow cooker to act as a trivet and place the wrapped meat on top.

Put the lid on, set to Medium and cook for 4½ hours, then remove from the cooker and the foil. (Alternatively, you can cook on a Low heat for 6–7 hours, or a High heat for 3½–4 hours, depending on the settings of your slow cooker.) Leave to rest for 10–15 minutes, then serve with the bread, salad and yogurt.

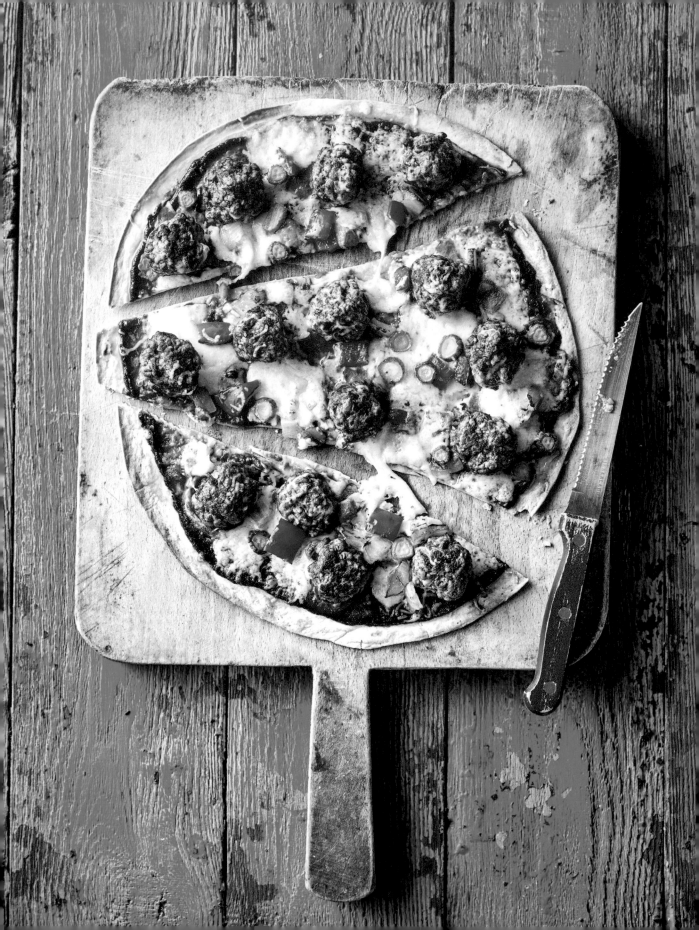

CHEESEBURGER PIZZA

🕐 **15 MINS** | 🍲 **15 MINS** | 🔥 **343 CALS** PER SERVING

Pizza can sometimes seem like the enemy when you're trying to follow a healthy diet, but by swapping a dense, carb-laden pizza base for a tortilla wrap you can eat it with a good conscience. Using some clever ingredients creates a classic cheeseburger taste, which feels like a real treat!

--- *Weekly Indulgence* ---

Meatballs only

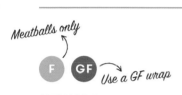

Use a GF wrap

SERVES 1

2¾ oz 5%-fat ground beef
pinch of dried oregano, plus extra
    for sprinkling
pinch of onion granules
pinch of garlic granules
salt and freshly ground black pepper
¼ onion, finely diced
¼ red pepper, finely diced
1½ tbsp tomato paste
1 tsp balsamic vinegar
1 low-calorie tortilla wrap
1 small pickled gherkin, thinly sliced
3 tbsp grated reduced-fat Cheddar
1¼ oz low-fat mozzarella

Preheat the oven to 425°F (fan 400°F). Line a baking tray with parchment paper.

Put the ground beef in a bowl with the oregano, onion granules and garlic granules. Season with salt and pepper, then mix well and divide into fifteen equal pieces, then roll them into meatballs. (You can freeze the meatballs at this point for cooking on another day.) Place the meatballs on the baking tray along with the diced onion and pepper. Cook in the oven for 5 minutes, then remove and set aside.

Turn the oven temperature down to 400°F (fan 375°F) and line a baking tray with parchment paper.

Mix the tomato paste with the balsamic vinegar and spread it over the wrap. Place the wrap on the lined tray.

Spread the cooked meatballs, onion and pepper over the wrap, then sprinkle with the gherkin slices. Cover with the grated Cheddar, then tear the mozzarella into small pieces and arrange on top. Sprinkle with a little extra oregano.

Cook in the oven for 7 minutes or until the wrap is crisp and the cheese is melted and golden brown.

Remove from the oven and serve.

HONEY *Chile* CHICKEN

🕐 **5 MINS** | 🗑 **25–30 MINS** | 🔥 **308 CALS** PER SERVING

Here at Pinch of Nom, we like to say that nothing is out of the question (in moderation). Using honey is a fantastic way to add natural, unrefined sweetness to your diet. Paired with the fiery warmth of chilli and balanced with the acidity of dark soy, this recipe is a tasty fakeaway option.

── *Weekly Indulgence* ──

Use GF soy sauce and stock cubes

F **GF**

SERVES 4

low-calorie cooking spray
1 lb 5 oz chicken thigh fillets (skin and visible fat removed)
2 tbsp runny honey
pinch of dried chile flakes
2 chicken stock cubes, crumbled
3 tbsp dark soy sauce
1½ tsp garlic granules

TO SERVE
2 radishes, finely sliced
2 scallions, trimmed and finely sliced
red chile, deseeded and finely sliced (optional)

Preheat the oven to 350°F (fan 325°F) and spray a baking dish with low-calorie cooking spray.

Place the chicken fillets in the baking dish.

Mix the honey, chile flakes, stock cubes, soy sauce and garlic granules in a bowl. Spread the mixture all over the chicken fillets and cook in the oven for 25–30 minutes until cooked through.

Remove from the oven and serve with radishes, scallions and red chile, if you like.

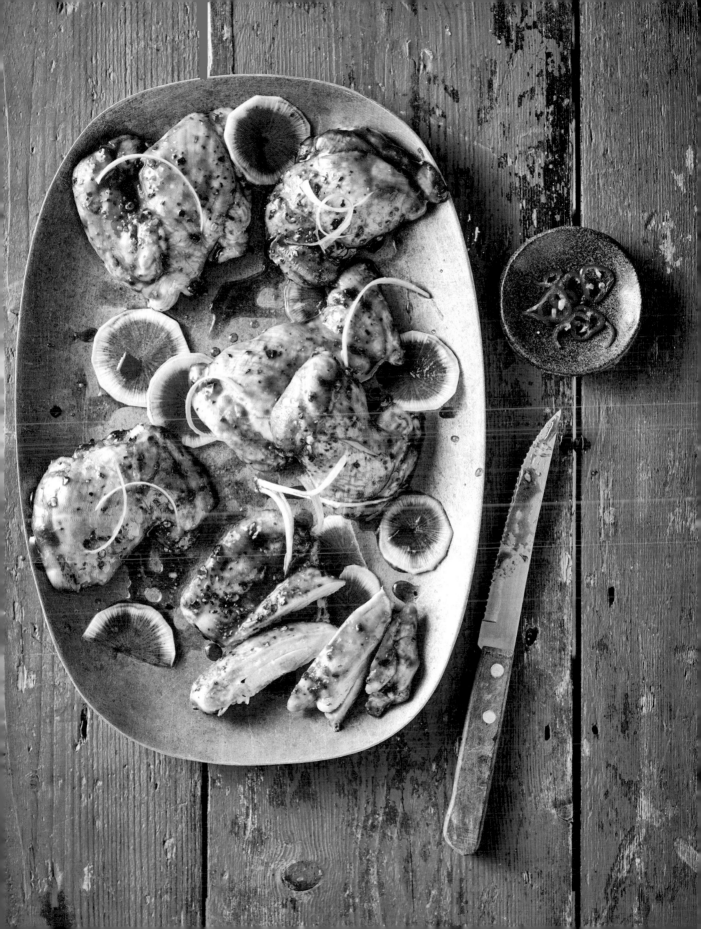

Diet Cola
CHICKEN

🕐 **10 MINS** | 🍲 **25 MINS** | 🔥 **217 CALS** PER SERVING

Diet cola may seem like a crazy ingredient, but trust us! This has become a classic Pinch of Nom recipe. When the majority of the liquid has evaporated (have patience – it will happen!) you're left with a sticky, sweet sauce that works perfectly with the balance and acidity of the vinegar tomato base. It is perfect served with freshly cooked rice for a Chinese fakeaway night.

———————————— *Everyday Light* ————————————

*Use GF soy sauce
and stock cubes*

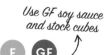

SERVES 4

low-calorie cooking spray
2 chicken breasts (skin and visible
  fat removed), diced
½ tsp Chinese 5-spice
sea salt
1 red onion, sliced
½ in piece of fresh ginger,
  peeled and finely chopped
3 garlic cloves, finely chopped
6 mushrooms, quartered
½ red pepper, deseeded and
  cut into strips
½ green pepper, deseeded and
  cut into strips
½ yellow pepper, deseeded and
  cut into strips
6 baby corn, halved lengthways
2 tbsp tomato paste
2 tbsp dark soy sauce
1 tbsp Worcestershire sauce
1 tbsp vinegar (such as sherry or rice)
1 (12 oz) can diet cola
½ chicken stock cube
1 chicken stock pot (such as Knorr
  concentrated chicken stock)
5 scallions, trimmed and
  roughly chopped

Spray a frying pan with low-calorie cooking spray and place over a low heat. Add the chicken, sprinkle with the Chinese 5-spice and season with salt. Stir and cook for a few minutes until the chicken has started to brown.

Remove the chicken from the pan and set it aside on a plate, add a few more sprays of low-calorie cooking spray to the pan, then add the onion, ginger, garlic and mushrooms and fry over a medium heat for 3–4 minutes until they start to soften, then add the peppers, baby corn, tomato paste, soy sauce, Worcestershire sauce and vinegar. Stir, then add the cola. Stir again and bring to the boil.

Crumble in the stock cube and the stock pot and simmer, uncovered, for 10 minutes. When the sauce has started to thicken and go a bit syrupy, return the chicken to the pan and stir in the scallions. Simmer for another 10 minutes. Check the consistency and if it's not quite thick enough, simmer for a bit longer, until the required consistency is reached, ensuring the chicken is cooked through.

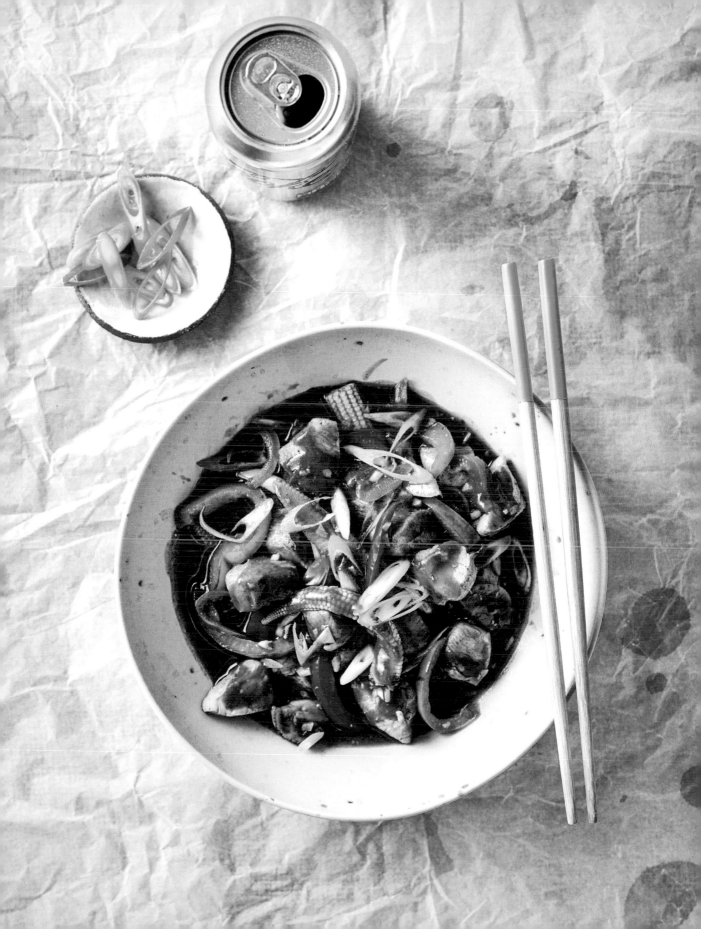

Chicken FAJITA PIE

🕐 **10 MINS** | 🍲 **45 MINS** | 🔥 **492 CALS** PER SERVING

Although it's slightly higher in calories than some of the other dishes in this book, this recipe is worth the indulgence every now and again. It is still lower in calories than a standard dish that uses a cheese sauce, and the smart ingredient swaps make this occasional treat worthwhile.

Special Occasion

(F)

SERVES 4

low-calorie cooking spray

3 chicken breasts (skin and visible fat removed), cut into thin strips

2 large yellow and/or red peppers, deseeded and thinly sliced

2 large onions, thinly sliced

1 tbsp ground cumin

½ tbsp ground coriander

1 tsp mild chile powder

½ tsp dried chile flakes (optional)

sea salt and freshly ground black pepper

1 (500g) carton passata (tomato puree; about 2 cups)

1 (14 oz) tin kidney beans in chili sauce

2 low-calorie tortilla wraps (cut to fit the tin if necessary)

2½ oz low-fat mozzarella

⅓ cup finely grated reduced-fat Cheddar

Preheat the oven to 400°F (fan 375°F) and line the base of a 9½ in springform cake tin with parchment paper.

Spray a large frying pan with low-calorie cooking spray and place over a low heat. Add the chicken strips and cook for 2–3 minutes. Add the peppers and onions to the frying pan, then add the spices, season with salt and pepper and mix well. Stir in the passata and kidney beans in chili sauce and leave to simmer gently for 15 minutes.

When the chicken is cooked, put a layer of chicken mix in the base of the lined tin, followed by a wrap, then another layer of chicken mix and another wrap, before finishing with a final layer of chicken mix. Top with chunks of the mozzarella and sprinkle over the grated Cheddar. Place in the oven and cook for 25 minutes until golden, then serve.

Tip
This is a SUPER adaptable recipe and works with whatever veg you've got in the fridge.

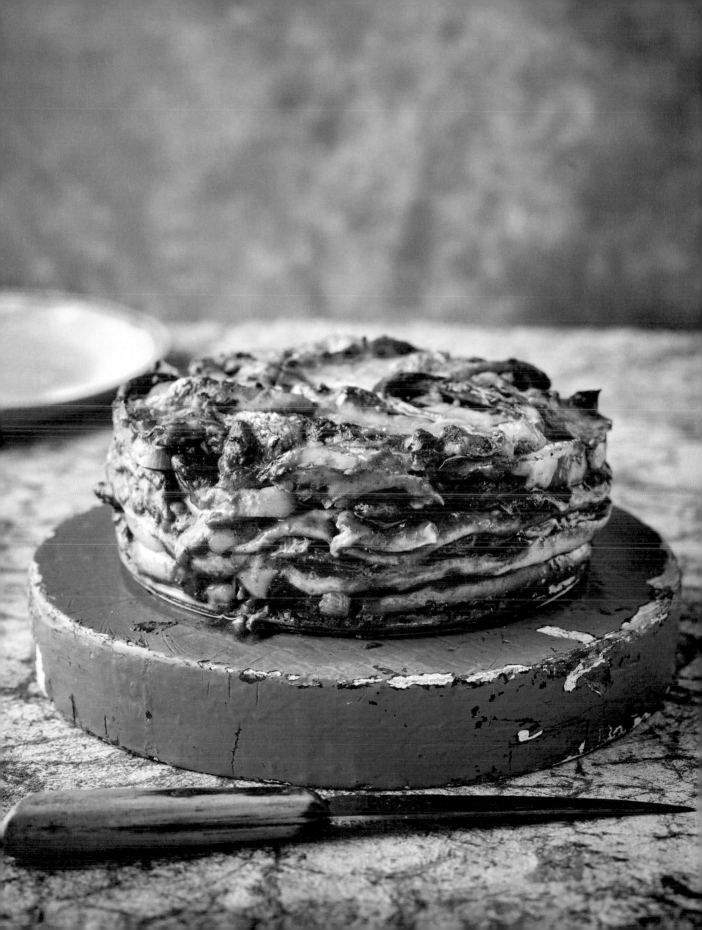

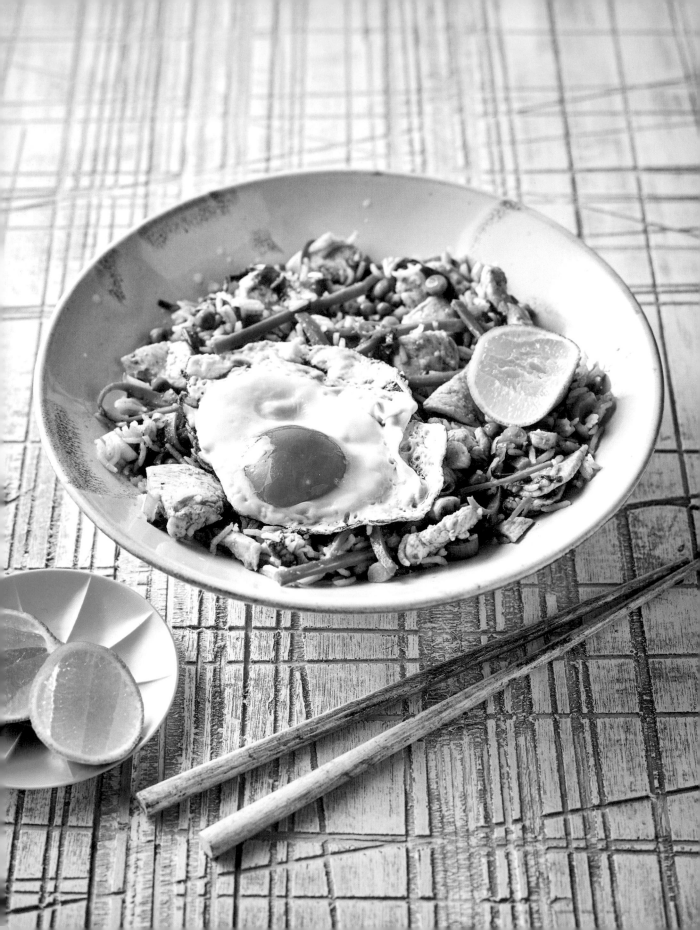

SINGAPORE FRIED RICE

🕐 **15 MINS** | 🍲 **20 MINS** | 🔥 **460 CALS** PER SERVING

This simple meal packs quite the flavour punch! Bulked out with cabbage, this rice dish is a great, quick recipe that really delivers on heat with the added curry powder. You can adjust the spice level to your preference, using whichever curry powder you like – mild, medium or hot. Trust us when we recommend putting a fried egg on top … when the yolk bursts and combines with the warming, filling mix below, it's just perfection.

Weekly Indulgence

Use GF soy sauce and stock cube

F **GF**

SERVES 4

1 cup basmati rice, rinsed and drained
1 chicken stock cube
low-calorie cooking spray
10⅛ oz chicken breast (skin and visible fat removed), cut into thin strips
6 scallions, trimmed and chopped
3 shallots, diced
1 medium carrot, cut into thin strips
2¾ oz pak choi or green cabbage, shredded
heaping ½ cup frozen peas
1 tbsp curry powder
1½ tbsp light soy sauce
1 tbsp fish sauce
4 medium eggs
½ lime

Cook the rice according to the packet instructions, using the chicken stock cube in the water, then drain and set aside.

Spray a wok or large frying pan with some low-calorie cooking spray and place over a medium heat. Add the chicken and cook for around 5 minutes, until cooked through, then remove from the pan and set aside.

Spray some more low-calorie cooking spray in the pan and place back over a medium heat. Add the scallions, shallots, carrot, pak choi or cabbage and the peas. Stir in the curry powder and cook for 5 minutes until the veg start to soften, but still have a bit of a crunch. Add the cooked chicken, rice, soy sauce and fish sauce and continue cooking and stirring until everything is piping hot and evenly coloured. (You can freeze the fried rice at this point for enjoying on another day.)

While everything is heating through, fry the eggs in a frying pan sprayed with a little low-calorie cooking spray, until they are done to your liking.

Finish the fried rice with a squeeze of lime, divide it among four plates and top each serving with a fried egg.

TURKEY KEEMA

🕐 **10 MINS** | 🍲 **25 MINS** | 🔥 **336 CALS** PER SERVING

Keema is ordinarily made with ground beef or lamb, rich with spices and ghee. This tasty, slimming-friendly alternative uses turkey. It's just as delicious and by using your own spices and fresh ingredients, it will still feel like an Indian takeaway night at home. Just what the doctor ordered!

Everyday Light

Use a GF stock cube
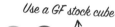

F **GF**

SERVES 4

1 red chile, deseeded (or leave the seeds in if you like more heat)
1 large onion, roughly chopped
¾ in piece of fresh ginger, peeled
2 garlic cloves, peeled
low-calorie cooking spray
1 lb 2 oz lean ground turkey breast
1 tbsp mild curry powder (or the spice mix below)
½ cup chicken stock (1 chicken stock cube dissolved in ½ cup boiling water)
1 (14 oz) tin chopped tomatoes
heaping 1 cup frozen peas
small handful of fresh cilantro, chopped, plus extra to serve
3 tbsp fat-free natural yogurt

FOR THE SPICE MIX (OPTIONAL)
1 tsp ground coriander
1 tsp ground cumin
¼ tsp ground turmeric
½ tsp ground cinnamon
¼ tsp smoked sweet paprika

TO SERVE
cooked basmati rice
1 lemon, sliced

Put the chile in a blender or food processor with the onion, ginger and garlic and blitz until smooth.

Combine all the spice mix ingredients, if using.

Spray a saucepan with low-calorie cooking spray and place over a medium heat. Add the ground turkey and cook for 5 minutes, breaking it up with a wooden spoon, then add the spice mix or curry powder and cook for another 2–3 minutes, until the meat is well coated. Add the onion, chile, ginger and garlic puree and cook for another 5 minutes. Add the stock and chopped tomatoes, bring to the boil and simmer for 10 minutes, until the sauce has reduced and thickened.

Stir in the frozen peas and chopped cilantro and cook for a further 3 minutes.

Remove from the heat, stir in the yogurt, and serve with basmati rice and lemon slices.

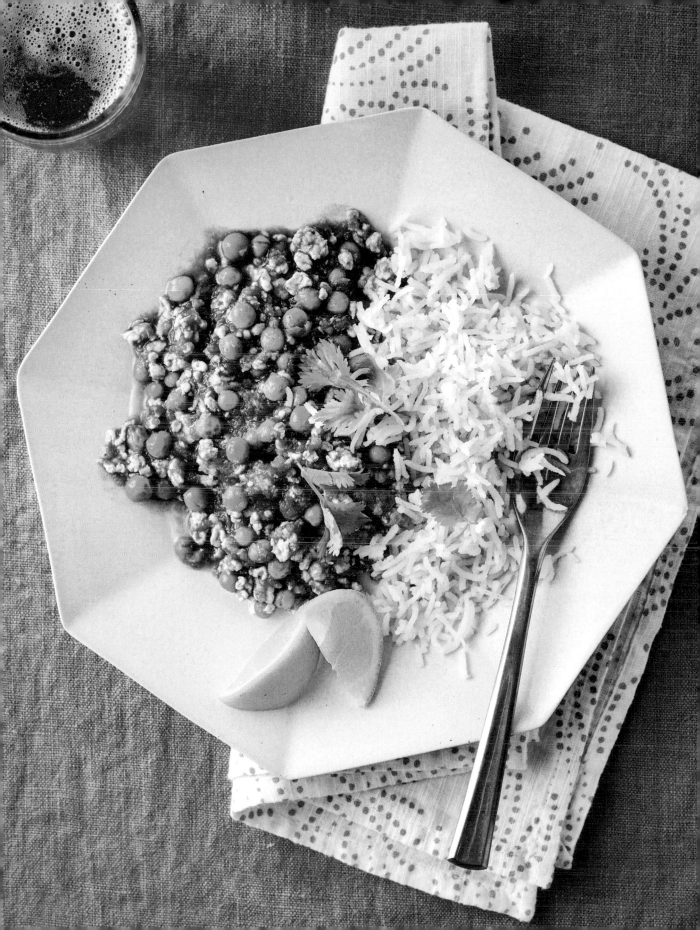

CHICKEN *in* BLACK BEAN SAUCE

🕐 **10 MINS** | 🍲 **10 MINS** | 🔥 **267 CALS** PER SERVING

We've given this classic Chinese takeaway dish the Pinch of Nom treatment, reducing the typical quantity of oil and calorific ingredients, while not sacrificing those authentic tastes of soy, miso and the depth of that spicy black bean sauce. A perfect Friday night craving sorted!

Everyday Light

F

SERVES 4

low-calorie cooking spray

1 lb 2 oz chicken breast (skin and visible fat removed), cut into strips

6 scallions, trimmed and chopped

3 garlic cloves, finely chopped

¾ in piece of fresh ginger, peeled and finely chopped

½ tsp Chinese 5-spice

¼ tsp dried chile flakes

½ (15 oz) tin baby corn, drained and each cut into 3

2¾ oz snow peas

½ red pepper, deseeded and sliced

½ green pepper, deseeded and sliced

2 tsp white miso paste

1 (14 oz) tin black beans, drained, rinsed and roughly mashed (make sure you use tinned, not dried)

4 tbsp light soy sauce

1 tbsp white rice vinegar

7 tbsp water

Sweet and Sour Crispy Asian Brussels Sprouts (see page 200), to serve (optional)

Spray a wok or frying pan with low-calorie cooking spray and place over a high heat. Add the chicken strips and stir-fry for 2–3 minutes until lightly browned, then add the scallions, garlic, ginger, 5-spice and chile flakes and stir well. Add the vegetables and stir-fry for another 3–4 minutes.

Stir in the miso paste and the crushed beans, followed by the soy sauce, rice vinegar and water. Bring to a simmer and cook for 2 minutes.

Check the chicken is cooked through and serve with Sweet and Sour Crispy Asian Brussels Sprouts, if desired, and/or rice or noodles.

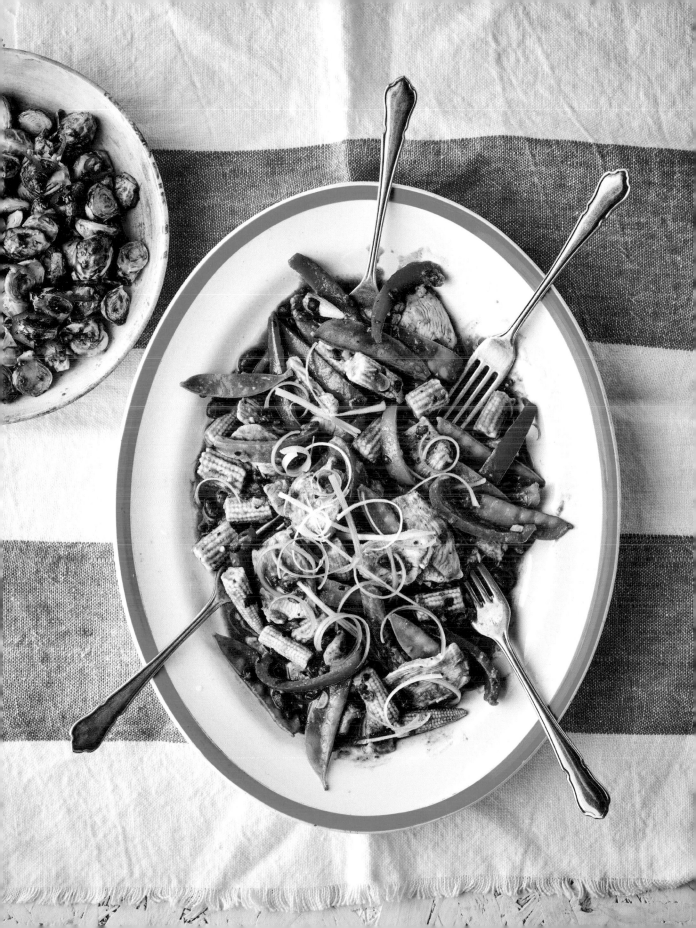

Veggie BURGERS

🕐 **15 MINS** | 🍲 **10 MINS** | 🔥 **118 CALS** PER SERVING

You can't beat a good veggie burger. The very best of them are substantial and tasty and, if you're a meat-eater, you don't even miss the meat. This is one of those great burgers. The addition of a small amount of Parmesan gives them a fantastic sharp, rich taste. Serve with a large salad and enjoy!

Everyday Light

Use GF buns

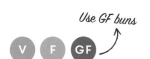

SERVES 4

8 oz medium potatoes, peeled and diced
sea salt
low-calorie cooking spray
2 garlic cloves, crushed
1 medium carrot, grated
½ cup trimmed and finely chopped green beans
½ cup finely chopped cauliflower florets
½ cup finely chopped broccoli florets
⅓ cup frozen peas
⅓ cup sweet corn kernels (tinned and drained, or frozen)
handful of fresh parsley, chopped
⅓ cup grated Parmesan (or vegetarian hard cheese)

TO SERVE (OPTIONAL)
4 whole-grain burger buns
lettuce leaves
Sweet Potato Rostis with Sour Cream and Chive Dip (see page 235)

Cook the potatoes in a pan of boiling salted water until soft, then drain well and mash with a hand-held masher or fork.

Spray a large frying pan with some low-calorie cooking spray and place over a medium heat. Add the garlic and all the vegetables (except the peas and sweet corn) and cook for 5 minutes, stirring so they don't start to colour. Add the peas and sweet corn and cook for another 2–3 minutes.

Mix the mashed potato and vegetables together in a bowl, then stir in the chopped parsley and Parmesan.

Divide the mixture into four equal pieces, and form each piece into a burger shape. (You can freeze the burgers at this point for cooking on another day. Thoroughly defrost the burgers before cooking.)

Spray a frying pan with some low-calorie cooking spray and place over a medium heat. Add the burgers and cook for 5 minutes or until they are golden brown on the bottom, then turn them carefully and cook for another few minutes. When the other side is golden brown, remove from the heat and serve the burgers on their own, in a whole-grain bun packed with lettuce, or with Sweet Potato Rostis (see page 235).

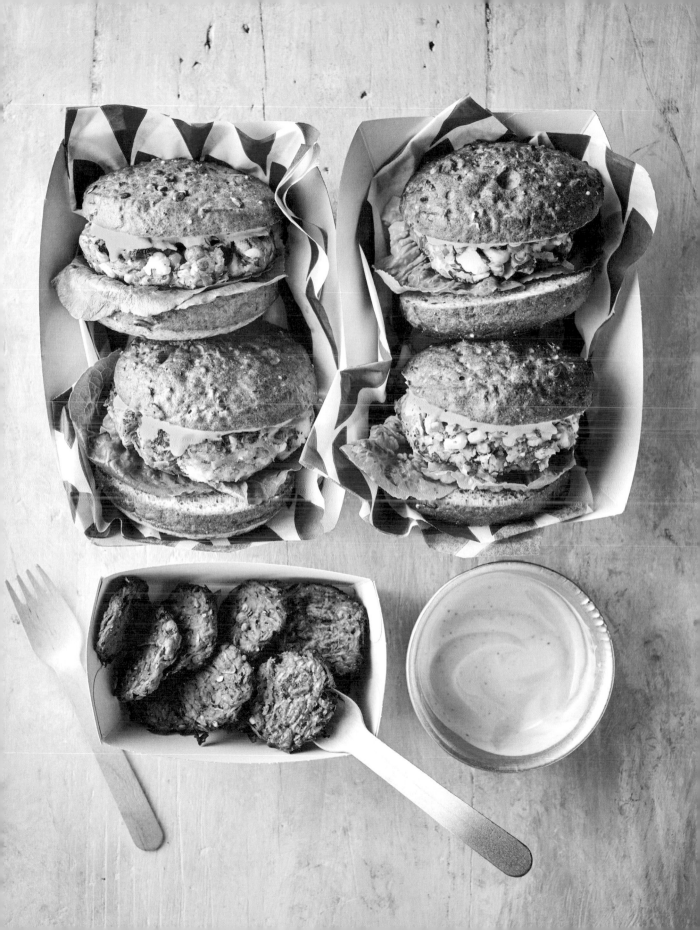

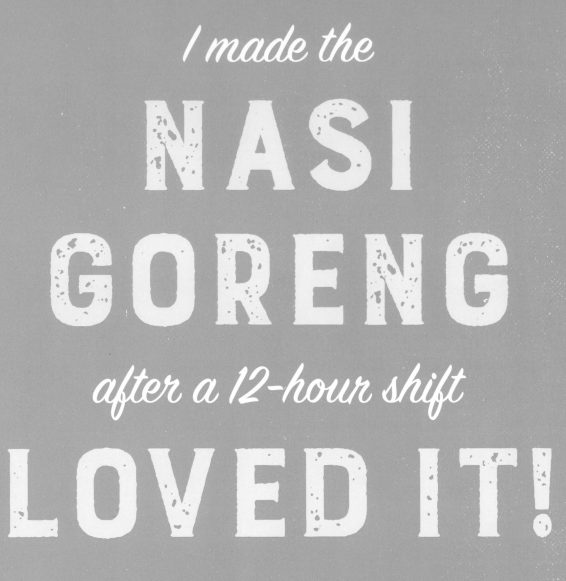

I made the
NASI GORENG
after a 12-hour shift
LOVED IT!

EMMA

"

I think **VEGETABLE BIRYANI** will be my new *fave* lunch: quick and easy!

CHARLENE

CHEESEBURGER PIZZA was *amazing*. I *love* that so many of the recipes are perfect for families.

CATHY

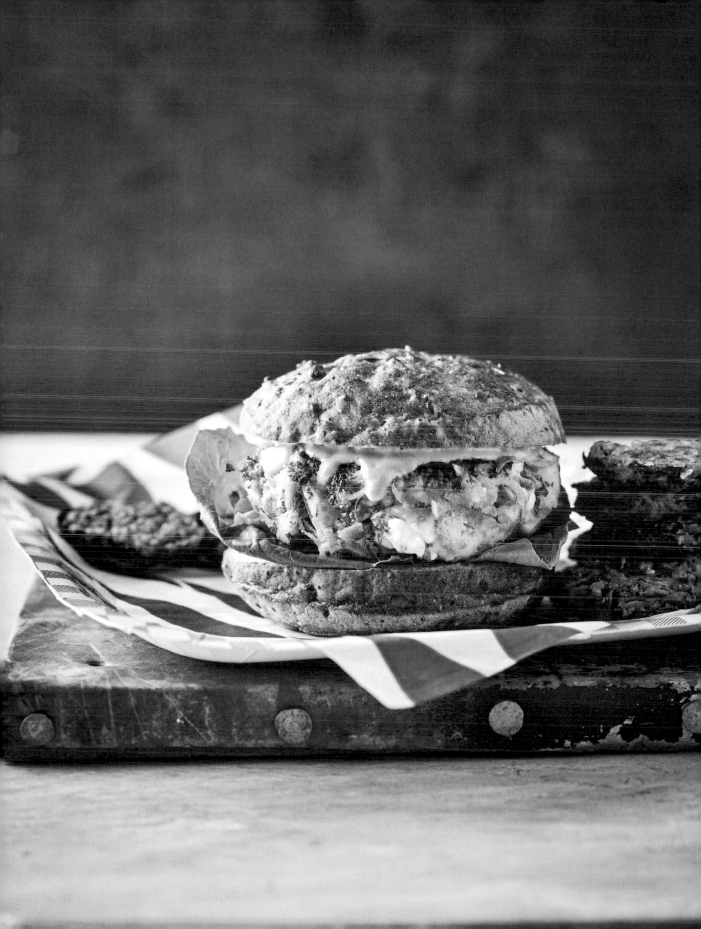

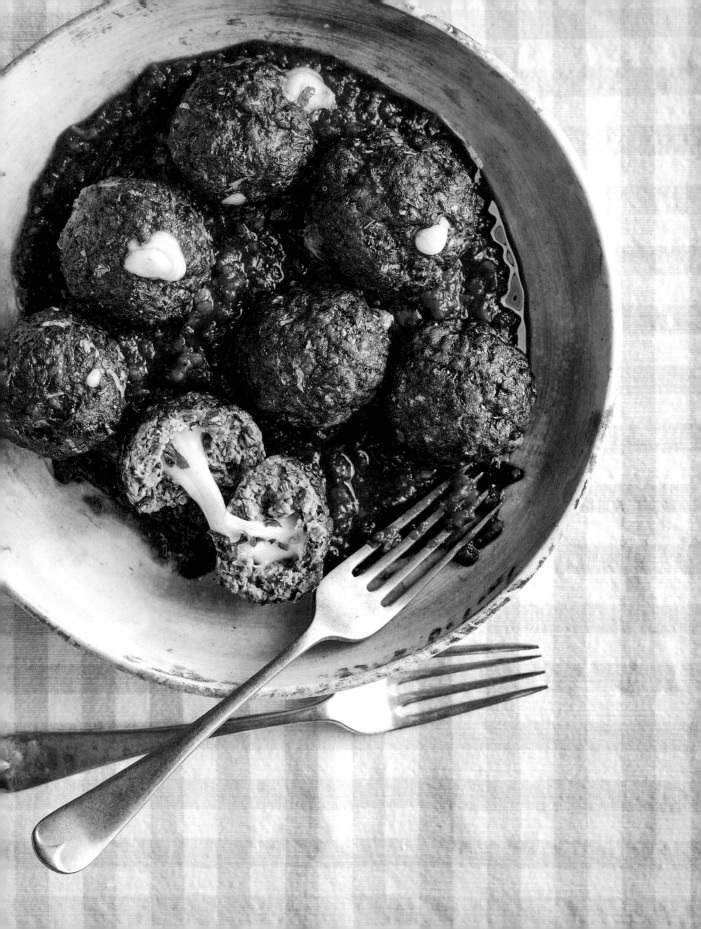

STUFFED MEATBALLS

🕐 **10 MINS** | 🍲 **25 MINS** | 💧 **283 CALS** PER SERVING

Delicious, rich tomato sauce and meatballs oozing with cheese … and this is slimming food? Yes! A small amount of mozzarella can go a long way into making these tasty meatballs seem like an absolute treat. So quick and easy to prepare, they can be whipped up on a weeknight for a busy family, with no fuss.

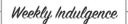

Weekly Indulgence

SERVES 4
(3 MEATBALLS EACH)

FOR THE MEATBALLS
1 lb 2 oz 5%-fat ground beef
1 tsp salt
pinch of freshly ground black pepper
½ tsp garlic powder
½ tsp dried oregano
½ tsp dried mixed herbs
1 medium egg yolk
handful of fresh parsley, chopped
2½ oz reduced-fat mozzarella, split
   into 12 equal pieces

FOR THE SAUCE
1 (14 oz) tin chopped tomatoes
¼ cup tomato paste
1 tbsp dried oregano
1 tsp onion granules
½ tsp dried basil
½ tsp dried parsley
1 medium carrot, finely chopped
1 celery stick, finely chopped
½ tsp red wine vinegar
sea salt and freshly ground
   black pepper

Preheat the oven to 400°F (fan 375°F). Line a baking tray with parchment paper.

Mix all of the meatball ingredients (except the mozzarella and half of the parsley) together in a bowl until well combined, then divide the meatball mixture into twelve equal pieces.

Enclose one piece of mozzarella in each portion of meatball mix. Firmly roll each one into a ball. Place the meatballs on the baking tray and cook in the oven for 15 minutes.

While the meatballs are cooking, make the sauce. Put all of the sauce ingredients in a pan, bring to the boil and cook over a low–medium heat for about 20 minutes.

Blitz the sauce with a stick blender, or in a blender or food processor until smooth, season to taste with salt and pepper, then return it to the pan. Add the baked meatballs to the sauce and stir well.

Sprinkle with the remaining chopped parsley and serve.

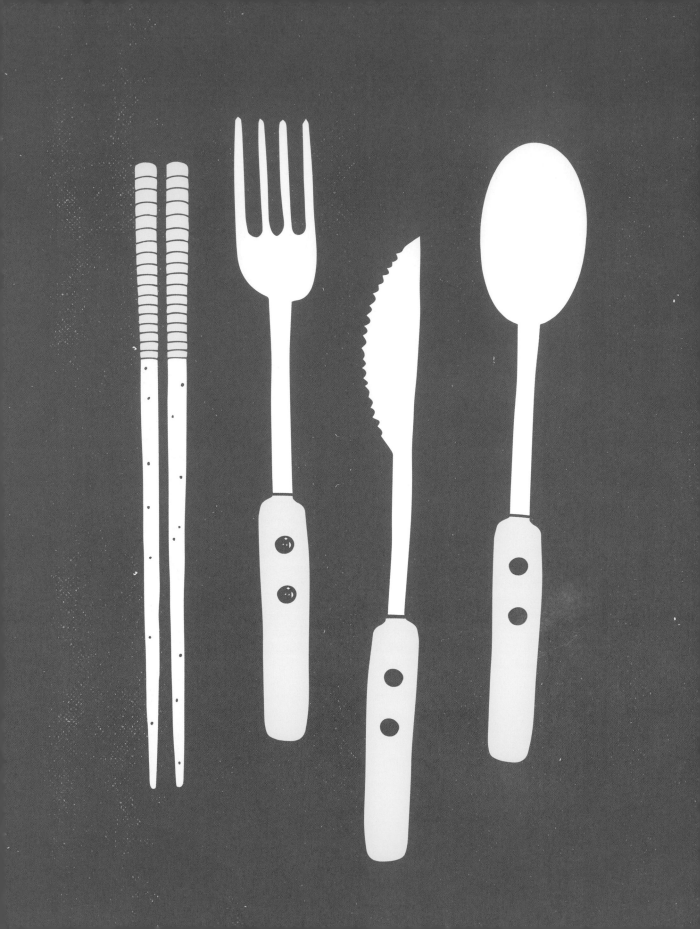

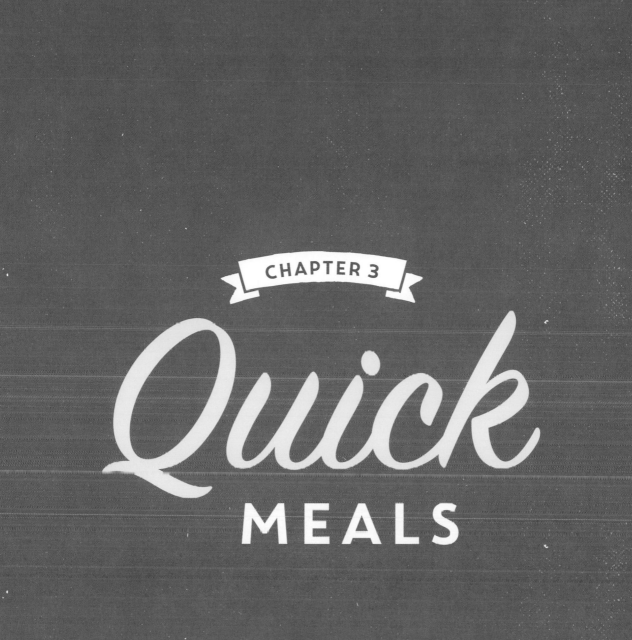

CHAPTER 3

Quick
MEALS

Rainbow COUSCOUS

🕐 **20 MINS** | 🍲 **NO COOK** | 💧 **280 CALS** PER SERVING

Couscous is a fantastically filling, low-calorie choice for a quick and easy meal. While pomegranate seeds may seem like an unexpected ingredient, their sweet tart flavour complements the salty feta, and the additional splash of red wine vinegar brings balancing acidity.

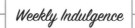

──────────────────────── *Weekly Indulgence* ────────────────────────

V

SERVES 4

1 cup couscous
1 vegetable stock cube
½ red onion, finely chopped
½ cucumber, diced
10 cherry tomatoes, halved
½ yellow pepper, diced
½ orange pepper, diced
1½ tbsp red wine vinegar
3 tbsp pomegranate seeds
handful of fresh mint, chopped
handful of fresh parsley, chopped
sea salt
6 tbsp crumbled reduced-fat feta
   cheese

Prepare the couscous according to the packet instructions, adding the vegetable stock cube to the water.

Stir all the veg into the couscous, then add the red wine vinegar, pomegranate seeds, chopped mint and parsley and mix well. Season to taste with salt.

Divide the couscous among four plates and sprinkle the crumbled feta equally over each portion.

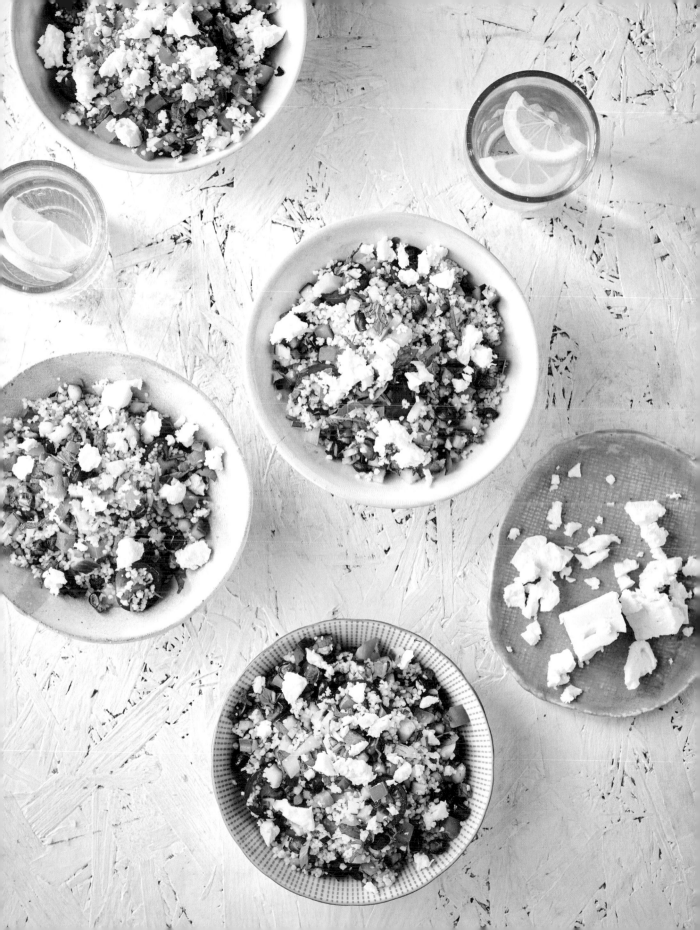

PIZZA-STUFFED CHICKEN

🕐 **10 MINS** | 🍲 **25 MINS** | 🔥 **388 CALS** PER SERVING

Chicken. And the flavours of pizza. Need we say more?! It's a match made in heaven. The chicken offers a protein-rich, filling alternative to calorie-heavy, dense dough bases. And a little reduced-fat melted cheese goes a long way.

───────────────── *Weekly Indulgence* ─────────────────

SERVES 4

4 chicken breasts (skin and visible fat removed)
20 thin slices of large mushrooms
½ red pepper, deseeded and cut into 20 thin slices
4 Canadian bacon medallions, each cut into 5 strips
½ red onion, thinly sliced
8 slices of tomato
¾ cup grated reduced-fat Cheddar
1 tsp dried Italian herbs
low-calorie cooking spray

Preheat the oven to 425°F (fan 400°F).

Take each chicken breast and make five cuts widthways across the breast, three-quarters of the way through from top to bottom. Be careful not to cut all the way through.

In each cut place the following: one slice of mushroom, one slice of pepper, one strip of bacon and a couple of slices of onion. Place on a baking tray and cook in the oven for 20 minutes, or until the chicken is cooked through.

When cooked, arrange two tomato slices on each breast and top each with one-quarter of the cheese and a pinch of the Italian herbs. Return to the oven and cook for another 5 minutes or until the cheese has melted and is golden brown.

Remove from the oven and serve.

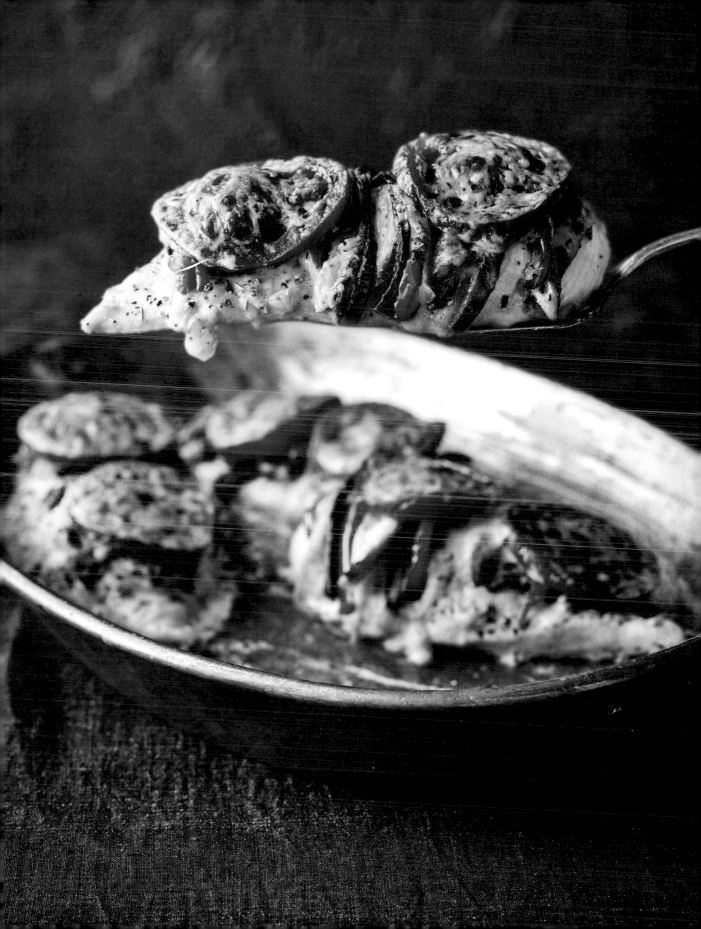

Moroccan
SPICED SALMON

🕐 **15 MINS** | 🍲 **20 MINS** | 🔥 **275 CALS** PER SERVING

Here at Pinch of Nom, our favourite phrase is "If it swims, it slims," with our fish dishes being our lightest main meals. This Moroccan-spiced salmon is a protein-rich, filling recipe that brilliantly combines the flavours of Morocco with the beautiful delicacy of the fish. It's also deceptively easy to cook, making it perfect for a quick yet sophisticated evening meal.

—————————————— *Everyday Light* ——————————————

SERVES 4

1 red pepper, deseeded
    and diced
1 yellow pepper, deseeded
    and diced
1 red onion, diced
low-calorie cooking spray
sea salt and freshly ground
    black pepper
4 skin-on salmon fillets
1 lemon

FOR THE SPICE MIX
2 tsp ground ginger
1 tsp ground cumin
2 tsp ground coriander
1 tsp ground cinnamon
1 tsp ground white pepper
½ tsp ground allspice
½ tbsp ground turmeric

Mix all of the spice mix ingredients together and set aside.

Preheat the oven to 400°F (fan 375°F).

Place the peppers and onion on a baking tray. Spray with some low-calorie cooking spray and season with salt and pepper.

Coat the top of each salmon fillet with the spice mix and place the fillets on top of the veg on the baking tray (you can keep any remaining spice mix in an airtight container for another time).

Cut the lemon in half lengthways and cut one half into eight slices. Arrange two slices on each piece of salmon and season with a little salt. Squeeze the remaining lemon half over the fish.

Place in the oven and cook for 20 minutes, or until the fish is cooked through.

Remove from the oven and serve the spiced fish fillets with the roasted vegetables.

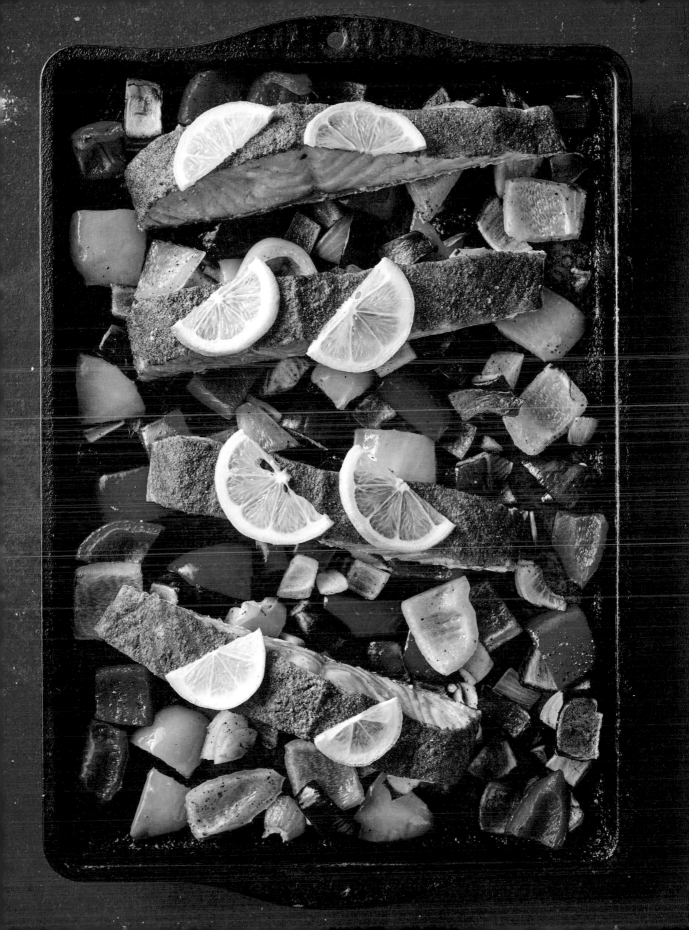

SMOKED SALMON *and* BROCCOLI QUICHE

⏰ **5 MINS** | 🍲 **30–35 MINS** | 🔥 **137 CALS** PER SERVING

The beautiful, delicate combination of broccoli and smoked salmon works wonderfully in this protein-rich quiche. A touch of seasoning and a generous sprinkle of scallions adds a punch of flavour to make this a recipe you'll make time and time again.

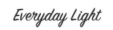 *Everyday Light*

SERVES 6

1 medium head of broccoli, cut into
   small florets
low-calorie cooking spray
2 scallions, trimmed and finely
   chopped
8 large eggs
2 tbsp quark or low-fat Greek yogurt
sea salt and freshly ground
   black pepper
4–6 slices of smoked salmon, cut
   into small pieces

Preheat the oven to 400°F (fan 375°F).

Steam or boil the broccoli florets for 3–4 minutes, then drain and pat dry with a paper towel. Set aside to cool.

Spray a frying pan with a little low-calorie cooking spray, place over a medium heat, add the scallions and fry for 2–3 minutes until softened.

Beat the eggs with the quark and a pinch each of salt and pepper in a medium bowl until smooth with no lumps.

Arrange the broccoli, smoked salmon and scallions in an 8 in round silicone mould or flan dish, then pour over the egg mix. Bake in the oven for 20–25 minutes or until set and golden on the top.

Remove from the oven and serve warm or cold.

Tip

A Pinch of Nom favourite, quark is an unflavoured soft cheese that gives a rich creaminess to recipes, while also being low in fat.

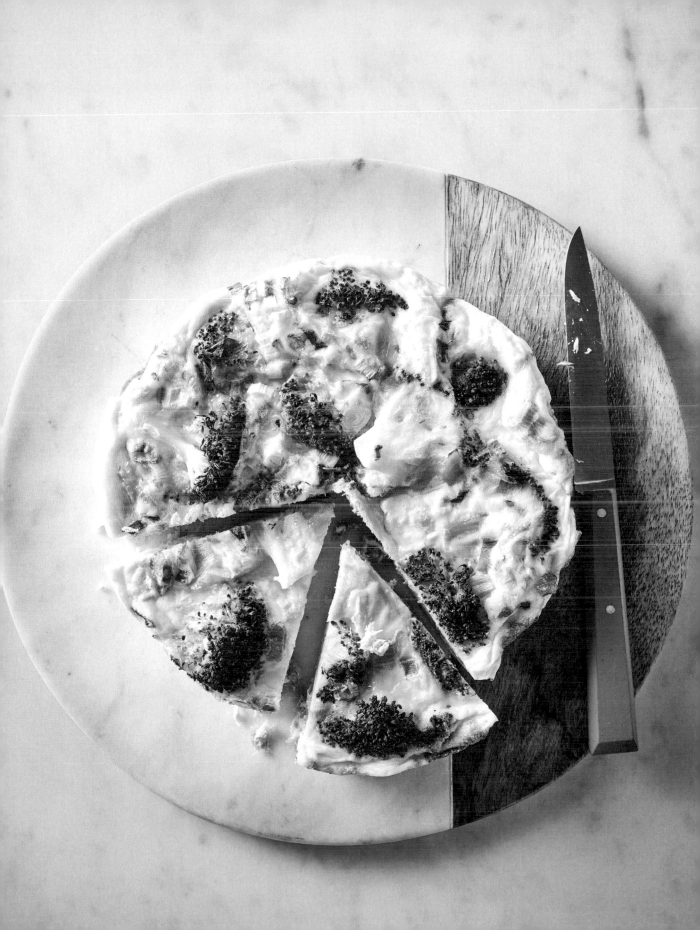

Coronation
CHICKEN

🕐 **10 MINS** | 🍲 **NO COOK** | 🔥 **329 CALS** PER SERVING

A British classic, this dish was prepared for the coronation of Queen Elizabeth II, and has thereafter been known as Coronation Chicken. The traditional recipe, usually rich with crème fraîche, can be high in saturated fats and calories, but using quark and fat-free yogurt (or all low-fat Greek yogurt, if quark is unavailable) re-creates that delicious, creamy taste without the high calorie count.

Weekly Indulgence

SERVES 2

¼ cup quark or fat-free Greek yogurt
scant ½ cup fat-free natural yogurt
½ cup grated firm mango
2 fresh apricots, stoned, peeled
   and chopped
pinch of granulated sweetener
1 tsp mild curry powder
1 scallion, trimmed and
   chopped
pinch of garlic powder
sea salt and freshly ground
   black pepper
1⅓ cup cooked chicken breast (skin
   and visible fat removed), diced
sliced brown bread, to
   serve (optional)

Mix the quark with the yogurt in a bowl, then add the grated mango, apricots, sweetener, curry powder, half the scallion and the garlic powder. Season with salt and pepper, mix well, then add the cooked chicken. Stir well, taste and add a little more salt if necessary.

Sprinkle the remaining chopped scallion over the chicken and serve.

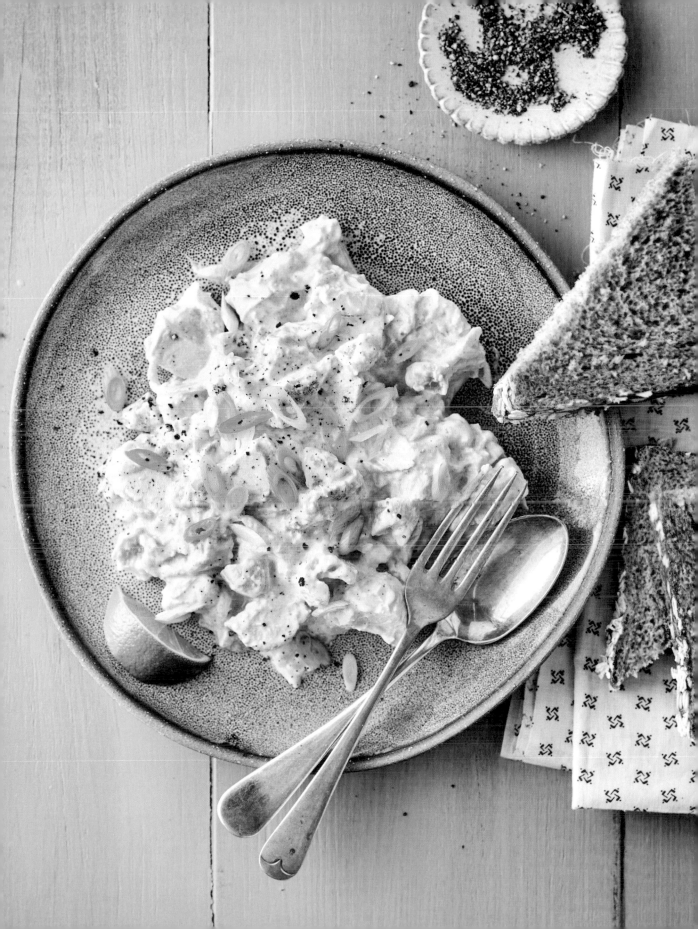

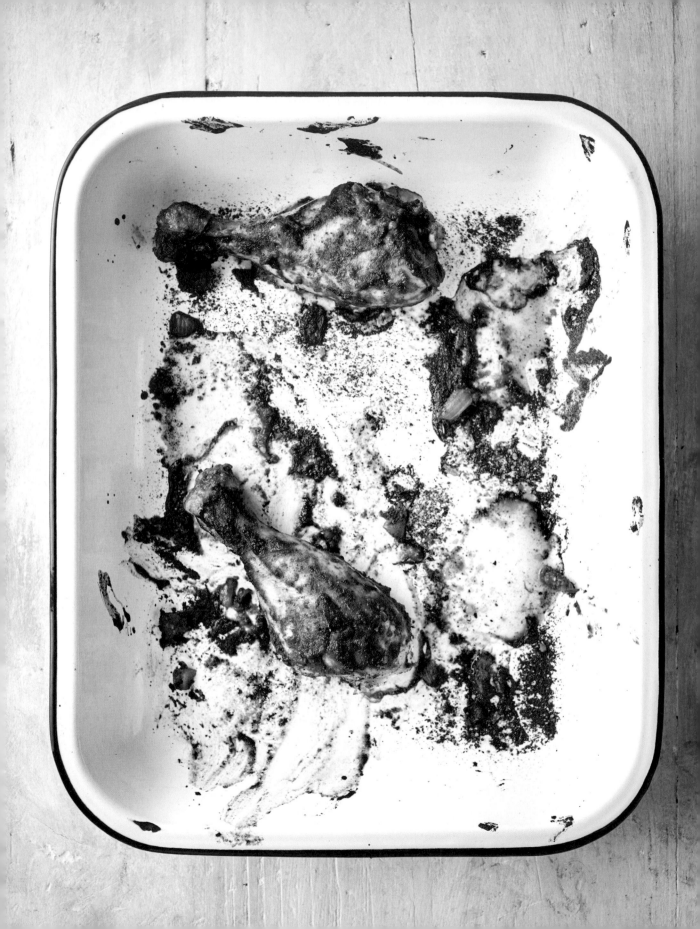

Made the
RAINBOW
COUSCOUS
tonight
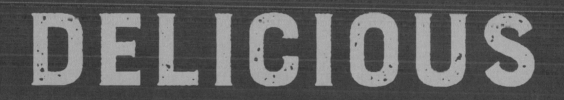
SO SIMPLE *and* REALLY
DELICIOUS

LISA

"

Made the CHICKEN and LEEKS in BLUE CHEESE SAUCE: dead easy and really *tasty*.

JULIA

The CHICKEN DIPPERS went down a storm. Even my anti-anything-healthy husband *loved* them.

ZARA

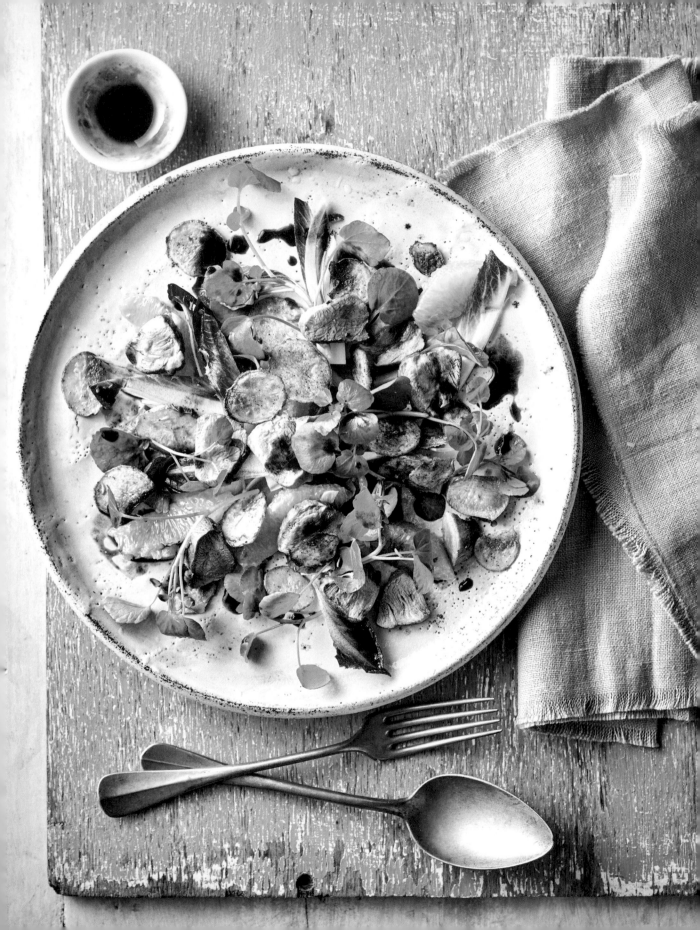

DUCK *and* ORANGE SALAD

🕐 **5 MINS** | 🍲 **20 MINS** | 🔥 **338 CALS** PER SERVING

This flavour combination is a true classic, but it can seem intimidating to the novice cook. This recipe keeps things really simple while still delivering the delicious taste of a rich duck breast and the acidity of the orange. The balsamic vinegar helps to balance out the flavours to make a delicious, easy evening meal.

Everyday Light

SERVES 2

low-calorie cooking spray
3½ oz new potatoes, thinly sliced
½ tsp Chinese 5-spice
1 duck breast (all skin and visible fat removed), cut in half lengthways
sea salt and freshly ground black pepper
2 large oranges, peeled and cut into segments (reserve any juice)
4 tbsp balsamic vinegar
lettuce leaves (as many as you like!)

Tip
Mixed leaves that have a bitter or peppery flavour, like watercress or arugula, work particularly well with this dish.

Preheat the oven to 400°F (fan 375°F).

Spray a baking tray with low-calorie cooking spray and spread the sliced potatoes out on the tray. Spray the potatoes with low-calorie cooking spray and sprinkle with the 5-spice. Place in the oven to cook for 10 minutes.

Meanwhile, spray a small frying pan with low-calorie cooking spray and place over a low heat. Season the duck breast and cook on one side for 7 minutes until really golden before turning and cooking for another 6 minutes.

After the potatoes have been in the oven for 10 minutes, turn them over, spray with more low-calorie cooking spray and put them back in the oven for a further 10 minutes until golden.

Remove the duck from the frying pan and set aside to rest.

Place half of the orange segments in the frying pan with any reserved orange juice and add the balsamic vinegar. Season with salt and pepper and reduce over a medium heat for 3–4 minutes. You should be left with a slightly thickened dressing.

Thinly slice the duck – it should be slightly pink in the middle. Put the lettuce leaves and potato slices in a dish with the duck and remaining fresh orange segments. Drizzle over the dressing and serve.

Chicken
DIPPERS

⏱ **10 MINS** | 🍲 **20 MINS** | 💧 **287 CALS** PER SERVING

This is a firm family favourite. Using whole-grain bread as a breadcrumb coating – and baking the chicken instead of frying it – makes this recipe the perfect healthy swap for discerning youngsters. These dippers are so tasty and crispy, you won't be able to tell the difference.

——————————————— *Weekly Indulgence* ———————————————

Use GF breadcrumbs

SERVES 4

8½ oz whole-wheat bread (stale bread works best)
½ tsp garlic salt
½ tsp garlic granules
½ tsp smoked sweet paprika
½ tsp dried oregano
1 large egg
4 chicken breasts (skin and visible fat removed), cut into strips
low-calorie cooking spray
reduced-fat mayo mixed with a little Sriracha, to serve (optional)

Preheat the oven to 375°F (fan 350°F) and line two baking sheets with parchment paper.

Blitz the bread into crumbs using a mini electric chopper or food processor. Place the breadcrumbs into a deep tub or bowl, add the garlic salt, garlic granules, paprika and oregano to the breadcrumbs and mix thoroughly. Beat the egg in a shallow dish.

Dip each strip of chicken into the egg and then place it into the breadcrumbs, ensuring that it is fully covered in the breadcrumbs. Place on one of the baking sheets. Repeat until all the chicken is coated. (You can freeze the coated chicken at this point for cooking on another day.)

Spray the breaded chicken strips with low-calorie cooking spray and pop into the oven to bake for 10 minutes, then remove from the oven, turn the pieces over, spray with low-calorie cooking spray again and return to the oven for another 10 minutes until golden and crispy.

Serve hot, with your choice of dip – we love Sriracha mixed with mayonnaise.

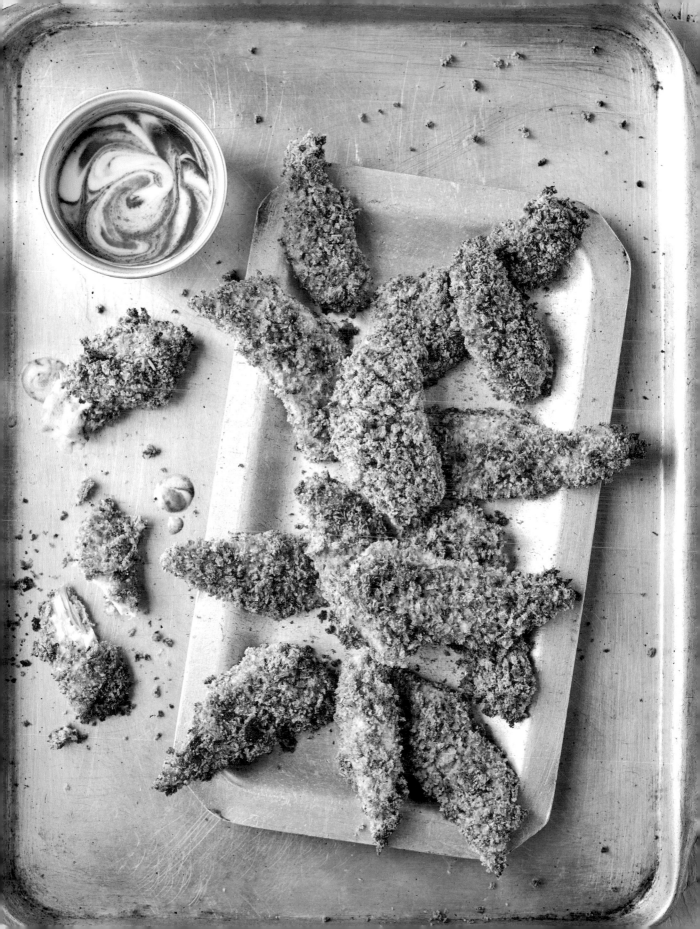

SHAKSHUKA

🕐 **10 MINS** | 🍲 **25 MINS** | 🔥 **242 CALS** PER SERVING

This North African dish is quite simply a tomato-based stew made with onions, garlic and peppers, with eggs poached in the mixture. It's a home comfort-style meal that's easy on the calories with a slight chile heat. Serve it with some new potatoes and green vegetables, or just on its own as a light meal.

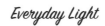

Everyday Light

SERVES 2

low-calorie cooking spray
1 onion, sliced
1 red pepper, deseeded and sliced
1 yellow pepper, deseeded
    and sliced
2 garlic cloves, finely chopped
    or grated
½ tsp ground cumin
¼ tsp mild chile powder
1 (14 oz) tin chopped tomatoes or
    cherry tomatoes
pinch of granulated sweetener
1 tsp lemon juice
3½ oz spinach
sea salt and freshly ground
    black pepper
handful of chopped fresh parsley
    or cilantro
4 medium eggs
Kickin' Cheesy Broccoli (see page
    210), to serve (optional)

Spray a large frying pan with some low-calorie cooking spray and place over a medium heat.

Add the onion and peppers and cook for 4–5 minutes until they have started to soften. Add the garlic and continue cooking for 4–5 minutes. (This should take 8–10 minutes in total.) Add the cumin and chile powder and stir for a minute or so, then stir in the tomatoes, sweetener and lemon juice. Cook for a couple of minutes, stirring occasionally.

Stir in the spinach, then turn the heat down to low, cover and cook for 5 minutes. Season to taste with salt and pepper.

Sprinkle half the parsley or cilantro over the tomato mixture, then make four wells in the mix and crack an egg into each one. Sprinkle the eggs with some salt and pepper, cover with a lid or foil and simmer over a low heat for 8–10 minutes if you like your eggs runny, or a bit longer if you prefer them firmer.

Remove from the heat, sprinkle with the remaining parsley or cilantro and serve.

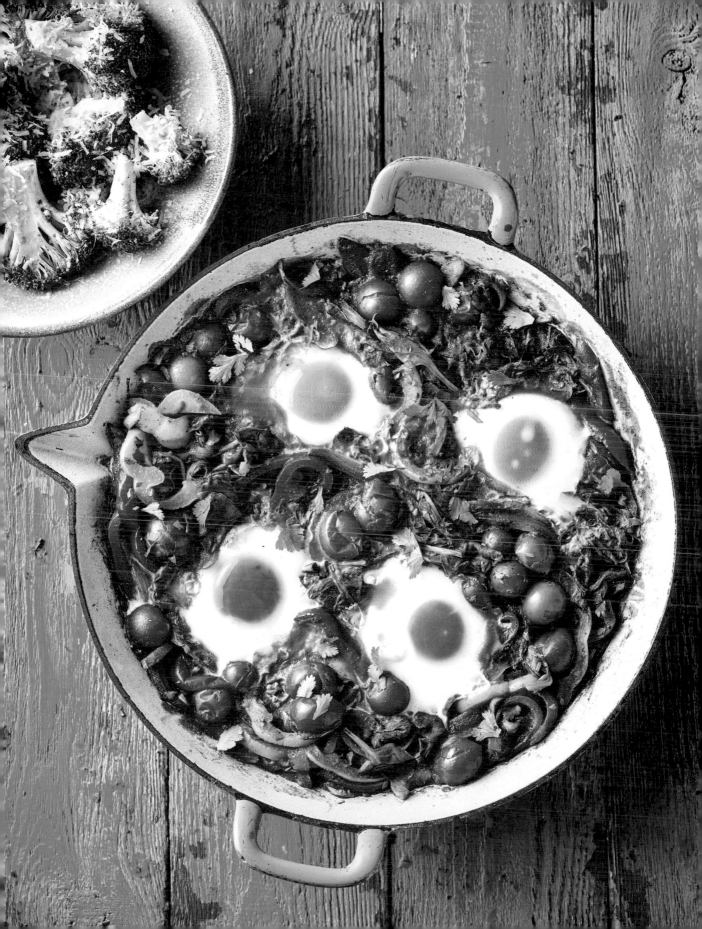

Pesto PASTA

⏱ **5 MINS** | 🍲 **15 MINS** | 🔥 **241 CALS** PER SERVING

A good, warming pasta dish is the perfect antidote to a bad day. Don't believe us? Just try this amazing recipe! Pesto can feel like such an indulgence, but if you leave out the oil and make it with fresh herbs you can re-create the fantastic flavour while minimizing the calories.

———————————————— *Everyday Light* ————————————————

F 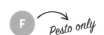 *Pesto only*

SERVES 4

11 oz dried pasta
1½ cups fresh basil
¼ cup snipped fresh chives
2 tbsp fresh parsley leaves
2 garlic cloves, peeled
1 tbsp Parmesan
sea salt and freshly ground
    black pepper
arugula, to serve (optional)

Place a large pan of water over high heat to boil for the pasta. Cook the pasta according to the packet instructions.

Meanwhile, put all the other ingredients in a mini electric chopper or food processor and blitz until the leaves are finely chopped.

Add 4 tablespoons of the boiling water which the pasta has been cooking in and blitz again, seasoning to taste with salt and pepper. This should create a glossy and bright green pesto.

When the pasta is cooked, drain and return it to the warm pan.

With the heat off, stir the pesto into the pasta. Serve warm.

Tip
You can freeze this pesto in an ice-cube tray to keep it for longer. It's so versatile, and perfect with meat, fish or veg!

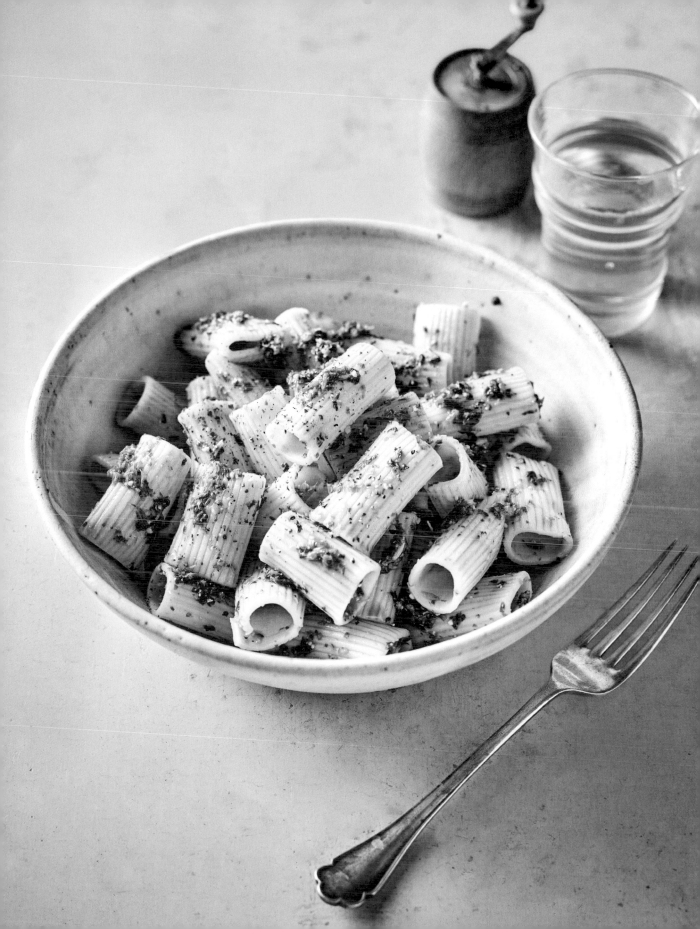

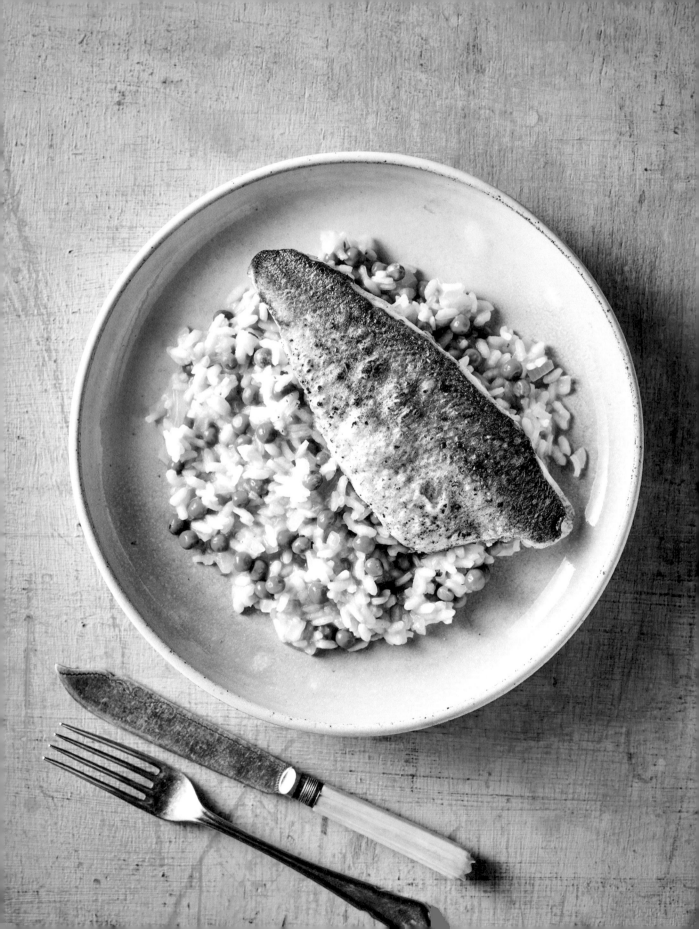

SEA BASS *and* MISO RISOTTO

🕐 **5 MINS** | 🍲 **25 MINS** | 🔥 **333 CALS** PER SERVING

Sea bass is a beautifully delicate fish that can often become overwhelmed by other flavours in a dish. However, this gentle miso risotto is the perfect accompaniment – it is flavoursome but doesn't take over the star of the meal, the fish.

Weekly Indulgence

SERVES 4

low-calorie cooking spray
1 large onion, finely chopped
1 garlic clove, crushed
heaping 1 cup Arborio risotto rice
3¾ cups fish or vegetable stock (1 fish or vegetable stock cube dissolved in 3¾ cups boiling water)
¾ cup frozen peas
1 tsp white miso paste
4 sea bass fillets

Spray a large frying pan with low-calorie cooking spray and place over a low heat. Add the onion and garlic and cook for a couple of minutes until soft but not browned. Stir in the rice.

Pour 1¼ cups of the stock into the frying pan and stir frequently for 10 minutes, until it has almost all evaporated, then add 1¼ cups more stock and continue to stir. When it has almost all evaporated add the final 1¼ cups of stock and turn the heat up to medium. Add the frozen peas and miso paste, stir well and cook for another 10 minutes.

Meanwhile, spray a separate frying pan with low-calorie cooking spray and place over a high heat. Add the sea bass fillets, skin-side down, and cook for 4 minutes, then turn them over and cook for a further 1 minute 30 seconds on the other side, or until the fish is cooked through.

The rice should now be tender, but with a slight bite. Divide the risotto among four plates and top with a sea bass fillet.

Tip
Why not try a drizzle of Sriracha over the top of the sea bass for an extra kick?

CHICKEN *and* LEEKS *in* BLUE CHEESE SAUCE

🕐 **5 MINS** | 🍲 **25 MINS** | 🔥 **214 CALS** PER SERVING

A good, smoky blue cheese can add a punch of flavour to any dish. The sauce in this chicken recipe is such a clever combination of ingredients that it will feel like an absolute indulgence. Tasty and hearty, this will become an instant family favourite.

Weekly Indulgence

Use a GF stock cube

SERVES 4

4 chicken breasts (skin and visible
    fat removed)
sea salt and freshly ground
    black pepper
low-calorie cooking spray
2 medium leeks, trimmed, washed
    and cut into thick slices
1¼ cups chicken stock (1 chicken
    stock cube dissolved in 1¼ cups
    boiling water)
5 tbsp low-fat cream cheese
¼ cup crumbled Danish blue cheese
Lazy Mash (see page 212),
    to serve (optional)

Preheat the oven to 400°F (fan 375°F). Line a baking tray with parchment paper.

Place the chicken breasts on the baking tray, season with salt and pepper, and cook in the oven for 20–25 minutes or until the chicken is cooked through.

Meanwhile, spray a frying pan with some low-calorie cooking spray. Add the leeks and cook over medium heat for 5 minutes, stirring often so they soften but don't colour. Pour the stock into the pan, bring to the boil and simmer until the liquid has reduced by about half, then stir in the cream cheese and Danish blue cheese. Stir, then simmer for a few minutes until the sauce starts to thicken.

Check the chicken. If it's cooked through, place each breast in a dish and divide the sauce equally over each chicken breast.

Serve with whatever you fancy – we like it with our Lazy Mash (see page 212).

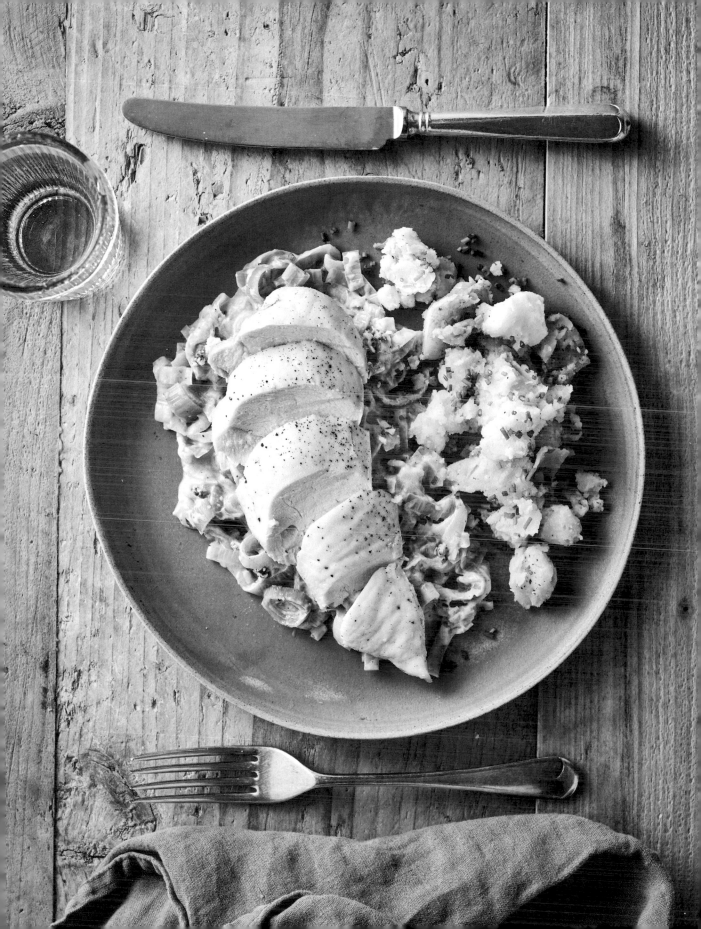

Sumac
LAMB CHOPS

🕒 **5 MINS** (PLUS CHILLING TIME) | 🍲 **10–15 MINS** | 🔥 **475 CALS** PER SERVING

Sumac is not an ingredient we see all that often. A versatile spice, with a tangy, lemony flavour, it's a fantastic seasoning for meat, and in particular, lamb. These beautiful chops taste like a takeaway dish and can be paired with our Easy Pilaf Rice with Chickpeas (page 209) for a delicious feast, conjuring dreams of a sunny holiday. They are perfect for summer barbecues.

──────────── *Special Occasions* ────────────

SERVES 4

1 tsp dried oregano
1 tsp ground cumin
pinch of ground cinnamon
1 tsp sumac
pinch of sea salt
scant ½ cup fat-free Greek-style
   yogurt
1 tsp tomato paste
8 lamb chops, all visible
   fat removed

Mix all the ingredients (except the lamb) in a non-reactive bowl, then add the lamb chops.

Cover the bowl and chill in the fridge for at least 1 hour, but preferably overnight. (Or you can freeze the marinated lamb in an airtight container for cooking at a later date.)

About 15 minutes before you wish to serve, take the lamb from the fridge and allow to come to room temperature. Fire up the barbecue or preheat the grill to maximum.

Grill on both sides until cooked – we like ours a bit rare. The cooking time will depend on the thickness of the chops, but they should take 5–7 minutes on each side.

Tip
You could serve with charred lemons. Place halved lemons cut-side down on the barbecue or a hot griddle pan. Cook for about 5 minutes.

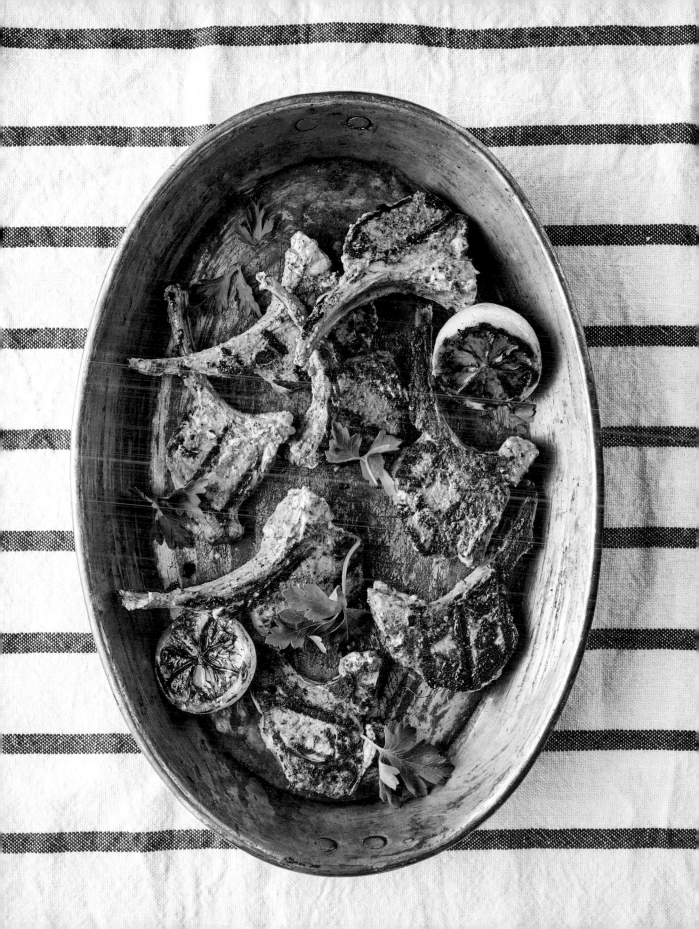

Cold Asian
NOODLE SALAD

🕐 **15 MINS** | 🍲 **3–5 MINS** | 🔥 **163 CALS** PER SERVING

This zingy, fresh salad is a perfect accompaniment to a main, but also works as a light stand-alone meal. The Sriracha adds warmth, and while fish sauce is not an everyday ingredient, it gives the salad its authentic Asian flavour. Lip-smackingly good!

—————————————— *Everyday Light* ——————————————

Use GF soy sauce

SERVES 4

FOR THE DRESSING
2 tbsp white rice vinegar
juice of 1 lime
1½ tbsp fish sauce
1 tsp granulated sweetener or sugar
2–3 drops of Sriracha, plus extra for
   serving (optional)
1 tsp light soy sauce

FOR THE SALAD
2 (1¾ oz) nests of fine rice noodles
   (you can use fine egg noodles
   instead, but this recipe works
   better with rice noodles)
2½ cups raw sugar snap peas, left
   whole or sliced lengthways
2 medium carrots, cut into thin strips
1 red pepper, deseeded and
   thinly sliced
6 scallions, trimmed and
   chopped
handful of fresh mint, chopped
½ handful of fresh cilantro,
   chopped

Cook the rice noodles according to the packet instructions, rinsing them in cold water once cooked, then drain.

Mix all of the dressing ingredients in a ramekin until the sugar or sweetener has dissolved.

Place all the salad ingredients in a bowl, add the drained noodles and the dressing, mix well and serve.

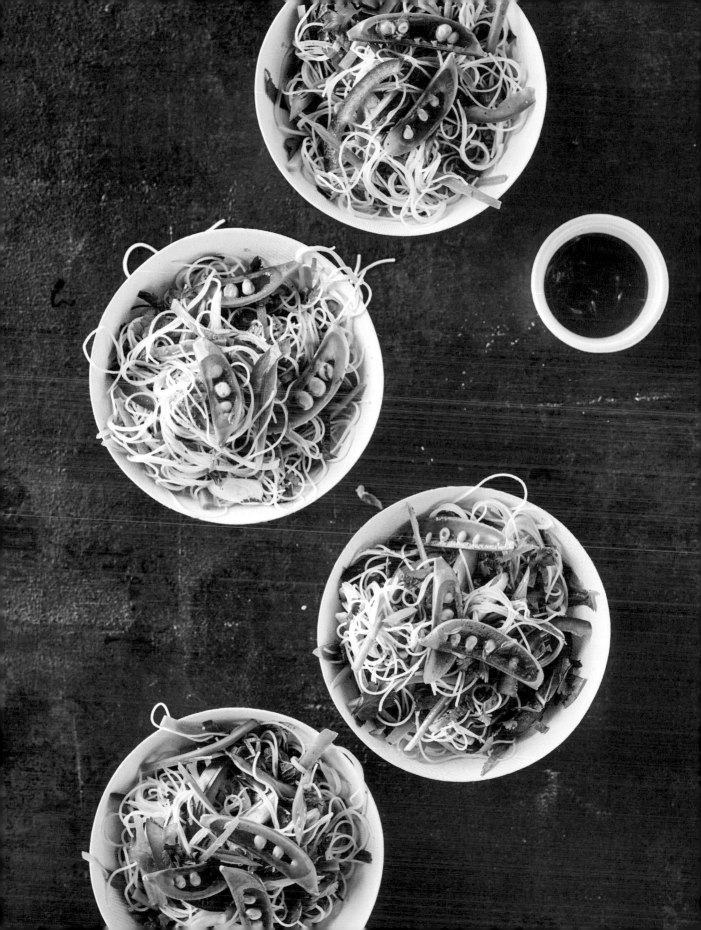

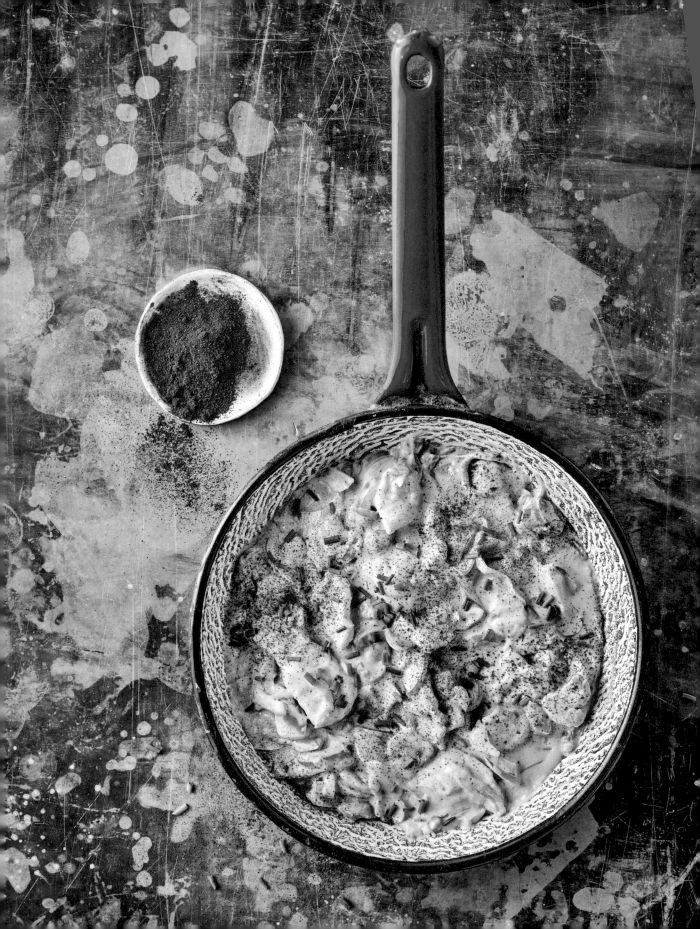

CREAMY GARLIC CHICKEN

🕐 **10 MINS** | 🍲 **20 MINS** | 🔥 **260 CALS** PER SERVING

This creamy garlic chicken recipe is rich and full of flavour, but it's not been anywhere near a jug of cream! Using low-fat cream cheese is a fantastic way to make this delicious meal and reduce the calories of the traditional, cream-based dish. This recipe will still seem like a treat and it's so simple to make. Serve with rice, pasta, fries, potatoes or anything you like.

Weekly Indulgence

Use GF stock cubes

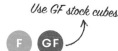

SERVES 4

14 oz chicken breast or thigh meat (skin and visible fat removed), thinly sliced
sea salt and freshly ground black pepper
low-calorie cooking spray
1 tsp white wine vinegar
1 tbsp Worcestershire sauce
1⅔ cups meat stock (1 beef stock cube dissolved in 1⅔ cups boiling water and mixed with 1 chicken stock pot such as Knorr concentrated chicken stock)
1 onion, thinly sliced
8 oz button mushrooms, thinly sliced
3 garlic cloves, thinly sliced or crushed
1 tsp Dijon mustard
12 tbsp low-fat cream cheese

TO SERVE
fresh chives, chopped
sweet smoked paprika (optional)

Season the chicken slices with a little salt and pepper, then set aside.

Spray a large frying pan with low-calorie cooking spray and place over a medium heat.

Add the chicken and quickly sear it on all sides, then remove the meat from the pan and set aside.

Return the pan to the medium heat. Add the vinegar to the Worcestershire sauce and deglaze the pan with the mixture, scraping and stirring the browned bits from the bottom of the pan – use some of the stock if you need to. When most of the liquid has evaporated, spray the pan with some low-calorie cooking spray. Add the onion, mushrooms and garlic and sauté for 5 minutes until they start to brown, then add the Dijon mustard and cook for a minute or two, stirring. Add the stock to the pan and simmer until reduced by half, then reduce the heat to low and stir in the cream cheese, making sure there are no lumps of cheese.

Return the chicken to the pan, stir well and simmer for 5–10 minutes until the chicken is cooked. If the sauce seems a little thick you can add some more water until it reaches the consistency you prefer.

Sprinkle with the chopped chives and paprika, if desired.

CAJUN *Dirty* RICE

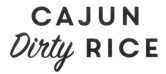

🕐 **10 MINS** | 🍲 **30 MINS** | 💧 **369 CALS** PER SERVING

This recipe was our first experience of "going viral" – the video for it has now been viewed over 5.2 million times! When we first posted it on Facebook, we never expected how many people would start to use Pinch of Nom recipes. Tried and tested by thousands of happy fans, this recipe is a quick and easy classic.

Everyday Light

Use a GF stock cube

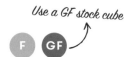

SERVES 4

1 cup plus 2 tbsp basmati rice
1 bay leaf
1 chicken stock cube
low-calorie cooking spray
14 oz 5%-fat ground beef
½ onion, finely chopped
4 Canadian bacon medallions, diced
2 tsp Cajun seasoning (or more, to taste)
dash of Worcestershire sauce
1 medium carrot, finely chopped
6 mushrooms, sliced
½ red pepper, deseeded and finely chopped
½ yellow pepper, deseeded and finely chopped
½ green pepper, deseeded and finely chopped
¾ cup beef stock (1 beef stock pot such as Knorr concentrated beef stock, dissolved in ¾ cup boiling water)
small bunch of scallions, trimmed and thinly sliced

Cook the rice according to the packet instructions, adding the bay leaf and chicken stock cube to the water before cooking. Set the rice aside once cooked.

Spray a frying pan with some low-calorie cooking spray and place over a medium heat. Add the ground beef, onion and bacon and cook for 3–4 minutes, stirring, until brown. Add the Cajun seasoning and Worcestershire sauce and stir, then add the carrot, mushrooms and peppers and pour in the beef stock. Cook for 3–4 minutes until the peppers start to soften.

Add the cooked rice and scallions to the pan and stir over a medium heat until all the rice is coated and it is warmed through. Taste and add some more Cajun seasoning if you prefer it spicier, then serve.

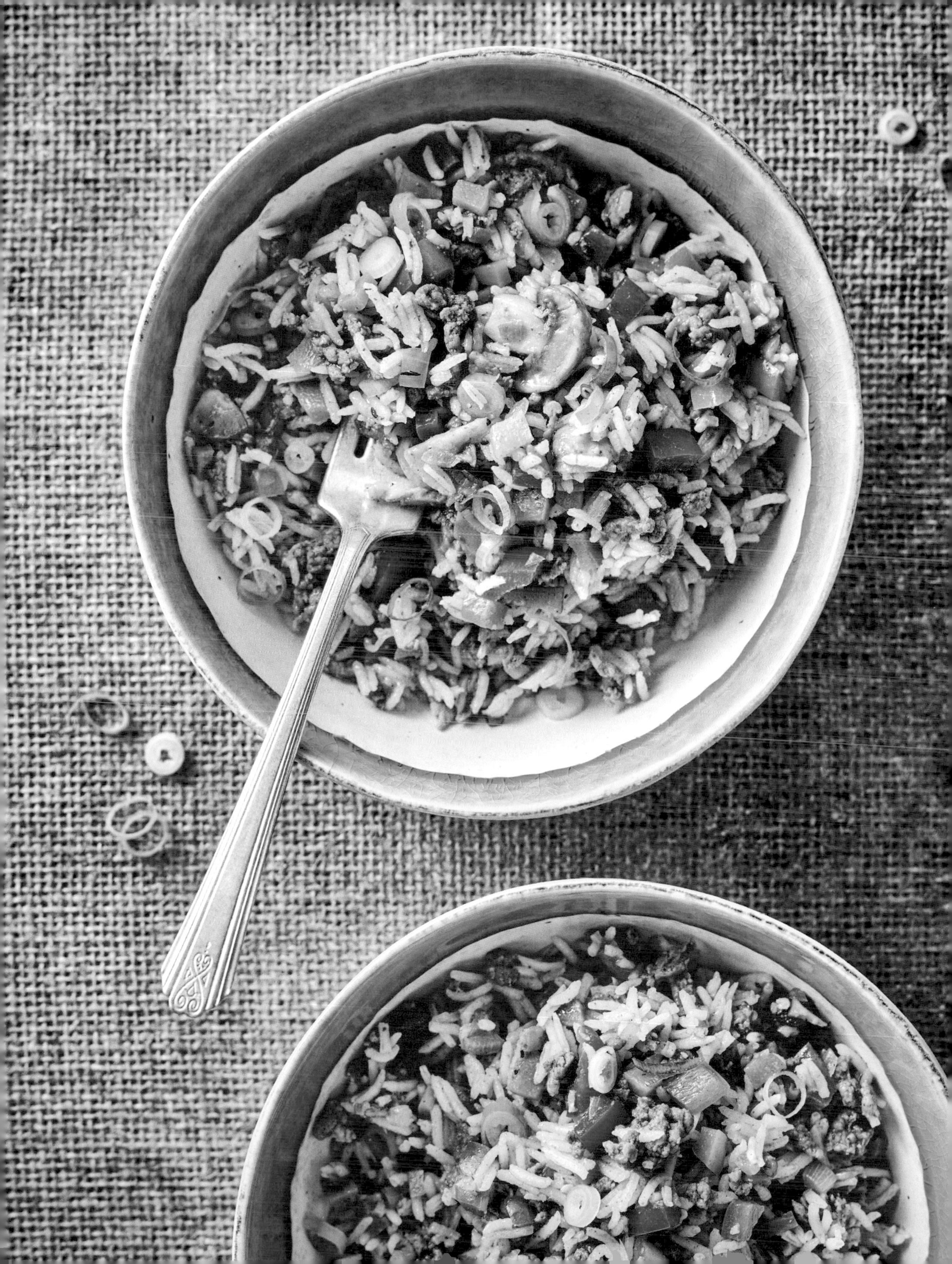

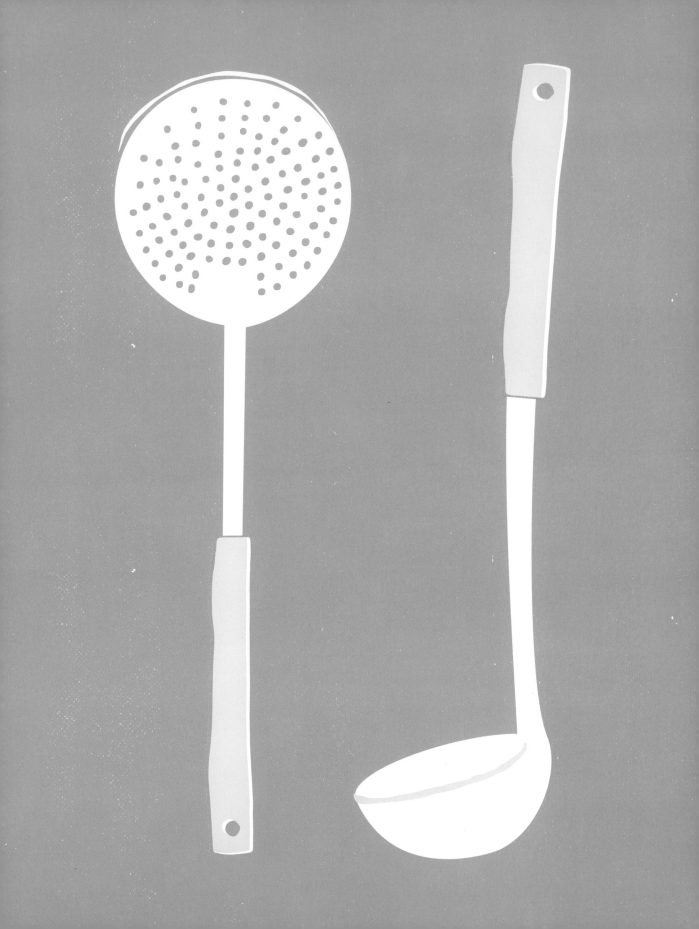

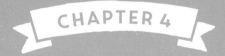

CHAPTER 4

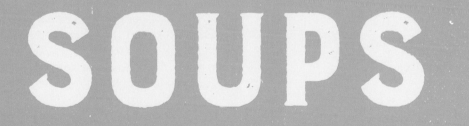

STEWS

and

SOUPS

VEGETABLE TAGINE

🕐 **10 MINS** | 🍲 **50 MINS** | 🔥 **198 CALS** PER SERVING

A wonderful Moroccan favourite, tagines are impressive and easy to make. The dried apricots and the spice mix add the really authentic flavours and you can leave it bubbling away to fill the house with the scent of Morocco as you prepare accompaniments. Delicious!

Everyday Light

Use a GF stock cube

(V) (F) (GF)

**SERVES 4
(GENEROUSLY)**

low-calorie cooking spray
1 large carrot, cut into
    chunky pieces
1 cup peeled rutabaga cut
    into chunky pieces
1 cup peeled parsnips cut
    into chunky pieces
6 shallots, peeled and
    halved lengthways
2 peppers, deseeded
    and diced
1½ cups peeled and
    deseeded butternut
    squash cut into
    chunky pieces
2 garlic cloves, crushed
1 tbsp ras el hanout
1 (14 oz) tin chopped
    tomatoes
1 cup vegetable stock
    (1 vegetable stock
    cube dissolved in 1 cup
    boiling water)
½ cup dried apricots, halved
1 (14 oz) tin chickpeas,
    drained and rinsed
sea salt

small handful of fresh
    cilantro, chopped

**FOR THE MOROCCAN
SPICE MIX**

2 tsp ground ginger
1 tsp ground cumin
2 tsp ground coriander
1 tsp ground cinnamon
1 tsp ground white pepper
½ tsp ground allspice
½ tbsp ground turmeric

Mix all of the spice mix ingredients together in a bowl and set aside.

Spray a large heavy-based pan with some low-calorie cooking spray and place over a medium–high heat. Add the vegetables and cook for 5 minutes until lightly browned (you may need to do this in batches).

When all the vegetables are browned, return them to the pan (if you cooked them in batches), add the garlic and cook for a few more minutes. Add the Moroccan spice mix and stir for a couple of minutes (keep any leftover seasoning in an airtight container for future use), then stir in the chopped tomatoes and stock. Bring to a simmer, stir in the apricots, cover and turn down the heat to low. Cook for 40 minutes, stirring occasionally.

Stir in the chickpeas, cook for another 5 minutes, then taste and season with salt if necessary.

Sprinkle with the chopped cilantro and serve.

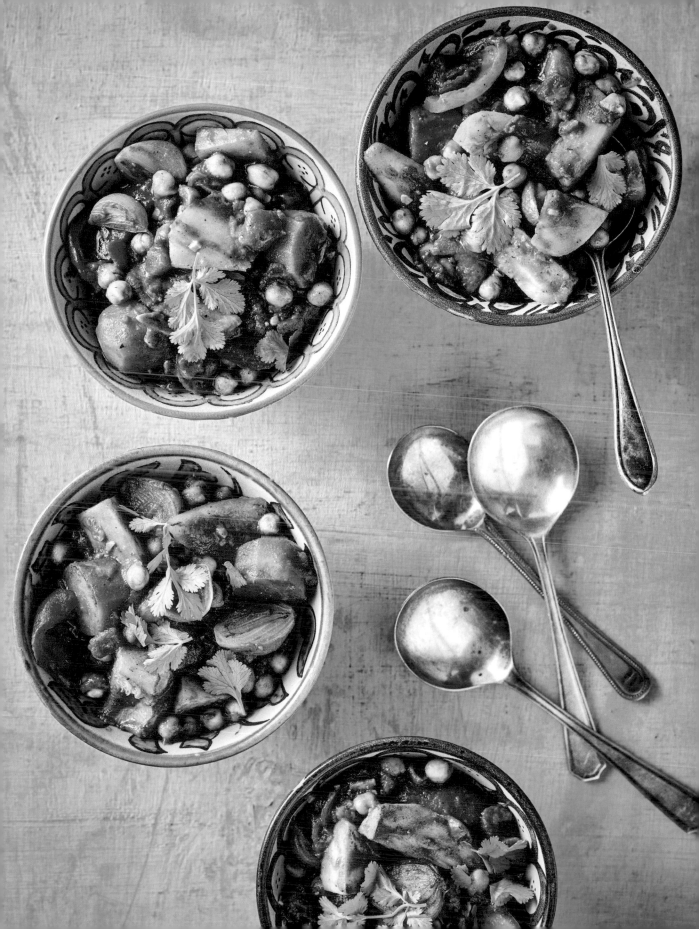

CAMPFIRE STEW

⏱ **30 MINS** | 🍲 **VARIABLE** (SEE BELOW) | 🔥 **409 CALS** PER SERVING

Sometimes there is nothing better to come home to than a warming, hearty meal. That's exactly what you get with this smoky campfire stew. A Pinch of Nom classic, we've included methods for using the oven, pressure cooker and slow cooker to cook lean ham or a piece of pork shoulder until it tenderly pulls apart. Bliss.

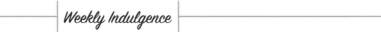

Weekly Indulgence

SERVES 4

1 (1 lb 10 oz) cured ham or uncured pork shoulder in one piece (all visible fat removed)
3 peppers (mixed colours), deseeded and chopped
2 onions, chopped
3 garlic cloves, crushed
1 tsp sweet smoked paprika
1 tsp ground cumin
1 tsp ground coriander
1 (16 oz) tin baked beans
1 (14 oz) tin chopped tomatoes
1 (14 oz) tin kidney beans, rinsed and drained
1 celery stick, chopped
2 large carrots, chopped
6–8 button mushrooms, halved
2 tbsp tomato paste
pinch of dried chile flakes
1 tbsp Worcestershire sauce
dash of hot sauce

OVEN METHOD

🍲 **3 HOURS**

Soak the ham joint overnight in cold water if necessary. Drain and rinse. (If using pork shoulder, there's no need to soak it.)

Preheat the oven to 375°F (fan 350°F). Keeping half of the chopped peppers to one side, add the remaining ingredients (including the rinsed gammon) to a casserole dish, stir well and cover with a tight-fitting lid.

Cook in the oven for 2–3 hours, stirring every 30 minutes or so and making sure there is enough liquid in the dish. After 2–3 hours, the meat should be starting to fall apart and sauce thickening. Remove the lid and, if necessary, continue cooking for a few minutes to thicken the sauce.

The meat should be soft and falling apart, but if it's not, shred it in the casserole dish with two forks and mix well. Around 15 minutes before the end of cooking, stir in the reserved peppers, then serve.

More methods on the next page …

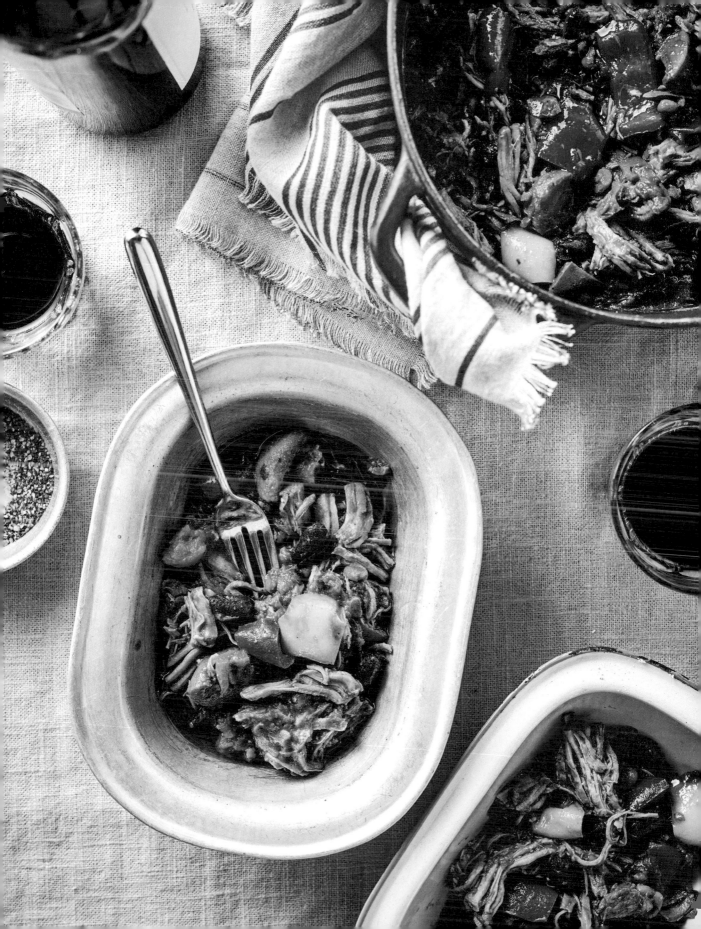

CAMPFIRE STEW ... *Continued*

ELECTRIC PRESSURE COOKER METHOD
🍲 **45 MINS**

Soak the gammon joint overnight in cold water if necessary. Drain and rinse. (If using pork shoulder, there's no need to soak it.)

Keeping half of the chopped peppers to one side, add the remaining ingredients (including the rinsed gammon) to the pressure cooker and stir well. Close the lid, turn the valve to "sealing" and pressure-cook on Manual/Stew setting for 40 minutes. Allow the pressure to release naturally (Natural Pressure Release/NPR).

Stir in the remaining peppers, close the lid, turn valve to "sealing" and cook on Manual/Stew until the cooker reaches pressure, then let the pressure release naturally.

The meat should be soft and falling apart, but if not, shred it in the pressure cooker with two forks and mix well before serving.

SLOW COOKER METHOD
🍲 **6–8 HOURS**

Soak the gammon joint overnight in cold water if necessary. Drain and rinse. (If using pork shoulder, there's no need to soak it.)

Keeping half of the chopped peppers to one side, add the remaining ingredients (including the rinsed gammon) to the slow cooker and stir well. Set the slow cooker to High, cover and cook for 6–8 hours. (You can leave it on longer.)

Around 30 minutes before the end of cooking, stir in the remaining peppers.

After 6 hours, check the consistency of the sauce and tenderness of the meat. The meat should be soft and starting to fall apart, and the sauce should be thickening. You can remove the lid and cook on High to finish the meat and thicken the sauce if necessary.

The meat should have broken up, but if it hasn't, shred it in the slow cooker with two forks and mix well before serving.

Cuban BEEF

🕐 **10 MINS** | **VARIABLE** (SEE BELOW) | 🔥 **279 CALS** PER SERVING

This dish combines the gentle heat of Cuban spices with tender beef,
which you can cook in the oven, or using a pressure or slow cooker.
Serve with rice or pasta for a hearty evening meal. *(Pictured overleaf)*

Using wine stock pots adds a special flavour while keeping the calorie count low.

──────────── *Weekly Indulgence* ────────────

Use GF stock cubes

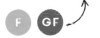

SERVES 4

1 (1 lb 2 oz) piece of stewing beef
   (all visible fat removed)
sea salt and freshly ground
   black pepper
low-calorie cooking spray
2 onions, sliced
1 cup beef stock (2 beef stock
   cubes dissolved in 1 cup
   boiling water)
1 (14 oz) tin chopped tomatoes
2 green peppers, deseeded
   and cut into strips
2 red peppers, deseeded
   and cut into strips
4 garlic cloves, crushed
2 tbsp tomato paste
1 tsp ground cumin
1 tsp dried oregano
½ tsp ground turmeric
2 bay leaves
1 tbsp fresh cilantro, chopped
2 red or white wine stock pots
1 tbsp white wine vinegar
cooked rice, to serve (optional)

STOVETOP OR OVEN METHOD
🍲 **2–2¼ HOURS**

Season the meat well with salt and pepper.

Spray a large frying pan with low-calorie cooking spray.
Brown the meat over a high heat then set aside.

Add a little more low-calorie cooking spray to the pan, then
sauté the onions for 3–4 minutes until they start to soften.

Add the remaining ingredients to the pan with the browned
meat and onions.

Bring to the boil then reduce the heat and simmer for
1½–2 hours or until the meat is tender. (You can also cover
the pan and cook in the oven for 2–2½ hours at 325°F, but make
sure your pan is ovenproof.)

Pull the meat apart with two forks – it should shred easily. If the
sauce is a little thin you can remove the lid to reduce the liquid.

Serve on a bed of rice or whatever you fancy.

More methods overleaf …

CUBAN BEEF ... *Continued*

ELECTRIC PRESSURE COOKER METHOD
🍲 1 HOUR 20 MINS

Season the meat well with salt and pepper.

Set the pressure cooker to Sauté/Browning, then spray it with a little low-calorie cooking spray. Add the meat and sauté for a few minutes on both sides until browned.

Add the remaining ingredients to the pressure cooker with the browned meat. Put the lid on the pressure cooker and pressure-cook on Manual/Stew for 1 hour, then allow the pressure to release naturally for about 15 minutes (Natural Pressure Release/NPR).

Pull the meat apart with two forks – it should shred easily. If the sauce is still a little thin, remove the pressure cooker lid and set to Sauté to reduce slightly.

Serve on a bed of rice or whatever you fancy.

SLOW COOKER METHOD
🍲 6–8 HOURS

Season the meat well with salt and pepper.

Spray a frying pan with a little low-calorie cooking spray and place over a medium heat. Add the meat and sauté for a few minutes on both sides until browned.

Add all the remaining ingredients to the slow cooker along with the browned meat. Set the slow cooker to High and cook for 6 hours, or on Medium setting for 8 hours.

Pull the meat apart with two forks – it should shred easily. If the sauce is still a little thin, remove the slow cooker lid and allow it to reduce slightly.

Serve on a bed of rice or whatever you fancy.

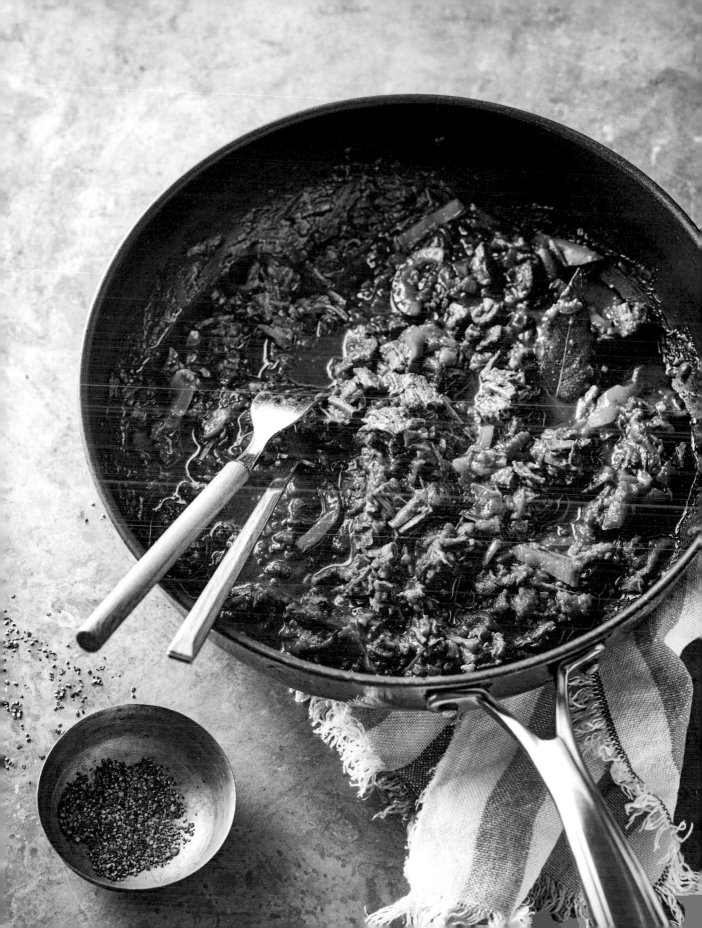

COCK *and* BULL

🕐 **10 MINS** | 🍲 **30 MINS** | 💧 **436 CALS** PER SERVING

You might not automatically consider cooking chicken and beef in the same dish. They become so tender and flavoursome together in this creamy sauce, but you could choose to use all steak or all chicken if you prefer. Family and friends will never guess that it's not made with cream!

──────────── *Weekly Indulgence* ────────────

Use GF stock cubes

SERVES 4

12 oz rump or sirloin steak (visible
    fat removed), cut into strips
12 oz chicken breast (skin and
    visible fat removed), cut into
    thin strips
sea salt
low-calorie cooking spray
1 onion, sliced
heaping 1 cup sliced mushrooms
½ tsp coarsely ground black pepper
2 cups beef stock (1 beef stock cube
    dissolved in 2 cups boiling water)
1 beef stock pot (such as Knorr
    concentrated beef stock)
13 tbsp low-fat cream cheese
handful of fresh parsley,
    finely chopped

Season the steak and chicken strips with a little salt, then spray a large frying pan with some low-calorie cooking spray and place over a medium heat. Add the meat and quickly sear on all sides, then remove from the pan and set aside.

Spray the frying pan with a little more low-calorie cooking spray and place it back over a medium heat.

Add the onion, mushrooms and black pepper and cook for 5 minutes until they start to brown. Add the beef stock to the pan and simmer until the liquid has reduced by half, then stir in the stock pot. Reduce the heat to low and stir in the cream cheese, making sure there are no lumps of cheese.

Return the meat to the pan, stir well, and simmer for 5–10 minutes until the chicken is cooked through. Taste and add a bit more black pepper if you like. If the sauce seems a little thick, add a little water until it reaches the consistency you prefer.

Top with the chopped parsley and serve.

Tip
For an extra indulgent treat, add a drop of brandy after you have browned the onions and mushrooms.

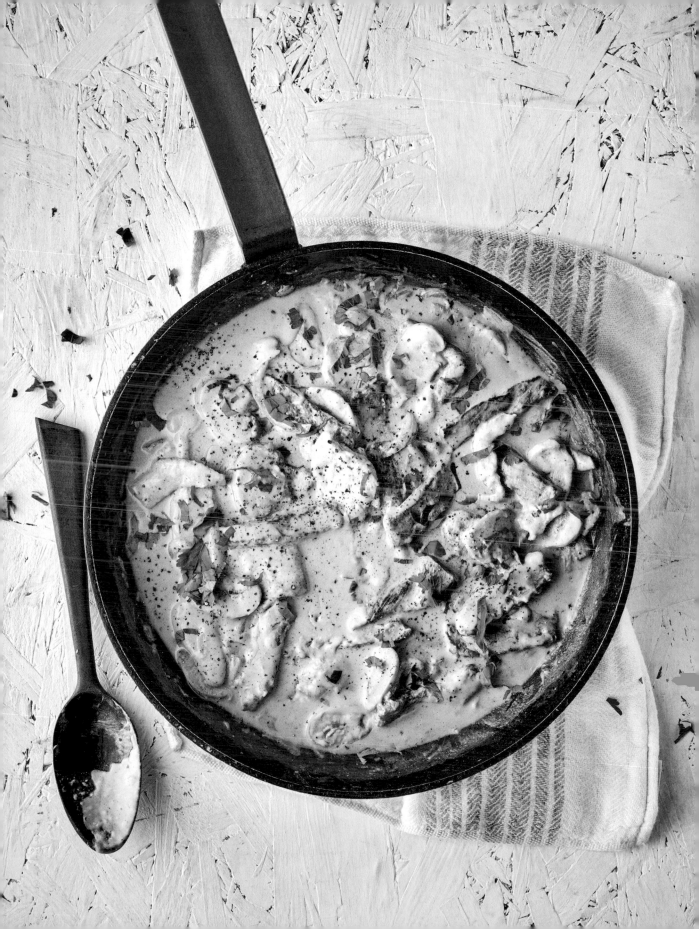

CAJUN *Bean* SOUP

🕐 **5 MINS** | 🍲 **VARIABLE** (SEE BELOW) | 🔥 **174 CALS** PER SERVING

This hearty, warming soup is packed with spicy Cajun flavours, kidney beans and filling vegetables. This wholesome soup feels like a meal in itself, and you can easily add some sliced cooked sausage or sliced bacon in for a meaty version – simply fry with the onions and garlic.

Everyday Light

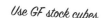
Use GF stock cubes
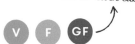

SERVES 6

low-calorie cooking spray
1 small red onion, diced
5 scallions, trimmed and chopped
2 garlic cloves, crushed
1 large zucchini, diced
2 red or yellow peppers,
    deseeded and diced
2 medium carrots, diced
generous handful of spinach (frozen
    is fine, but double quantity)
1 (14 oz) tin chopped tomatoes
1 (500g) carton passata (tomato
    puree; about 2 cups)
2 tbsp tomato paste
2¼ cups vegetable stock (2 vegetable
    stock cubes dissolved in 2¼ cups
    boiling water)
1–2 tbsp Cajun seasoning (to taste)
1 tbsp Worcestershire sauce (or
    vegetarian alternative like Biona
    Organic Worcestershire sauce)
1 tbsp white wine vinegar
1 bay leaf
1 (14 oz) tin red kidney beans,
    drained and rinsed
1 (14 oz) tin chickpeas, drained
    and rinsed
freshly ground black pepper

STOVETOP METHOD
🍲 **50 MINS**

Spray a large frying pan with low-calorie cooking spray and place over a medium heat. Add the onion, scallions and garlic and sauté for 4–5 minutes until softened.

Add the remaining ingredients (apart from the beans, chickpeas and black pepper), stir well and bring to the boil, then simmer for 30 minutes.

Add the kidney beans and chickpeas. Taste and season with pepper to taste. You can also add a little more Cajun seasoning if you need to.

Cook for another 15 minutes or so, remove the bay leaf, then serve.

More methods overleaf ...

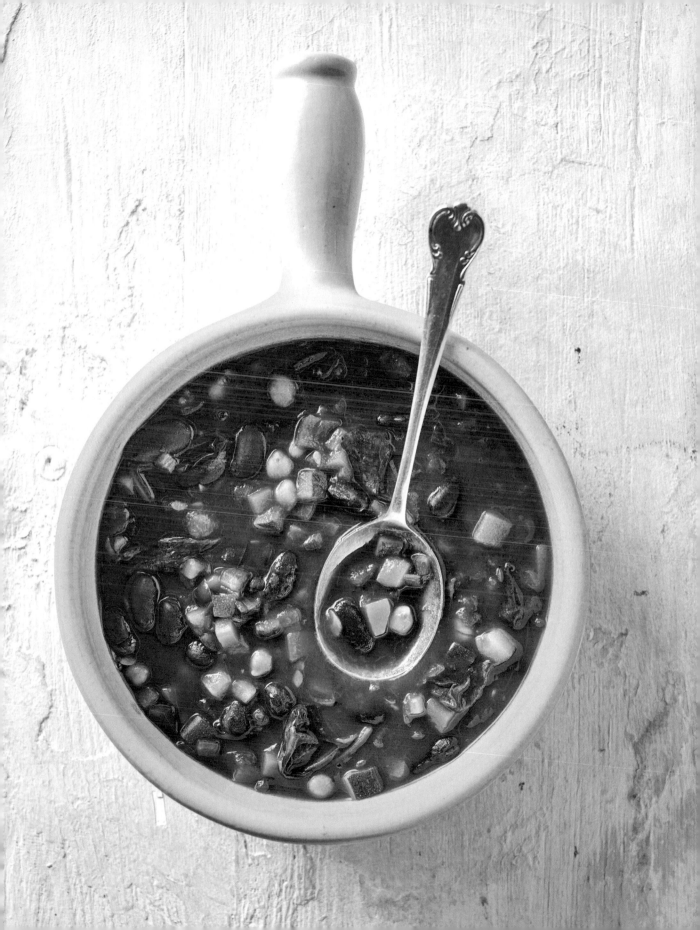

CAJUN BEAN SOUP ... *Continued*

ELECTRIC PRESSURE COOKER METHOD
🍲 30 MINS

Set the pressure cooker to Sauté/Browning, spray the inside with low-calorie cooking spray and cook the onion, scallions and garlic for 3–4 minutes until they start to soften.

Add the remaining ingredients (apart from the beans, chickpeas and black pepper) and stir well. Pressure-cook on Manual/Stew for 20 minutes. Allow the pressure to release naturally (Natural Pressure Release/NPR).

Add the kidney beans and chickpeas. Taste and add some black pepper to taste. You can also add a little more Cajun seasoning if you need to.

Set the pressure cooker to Sauté for another 5 minutes or so, remove the bay leaf, then serve.

SLOW COOKER METHOD
🍲 4 HOURS 10 MINS

Spray a large frying pan with low-calorie cooking spray and place over a medium heat. Add the onion, scallions and garlic and sauté for 4–5 minutes until softened.

Add the remaining ingredients (apart from the beans, chickpeas and black pepper), stir well and bring to the boil, then pour the soup into a slow cooker and cook on Medium setting for 3 hours.

After 3 hours, add the kidney beans and chickpeas. Add some black pepper to taste, and a little more Cajun seasoning if you like. Cook for another hour or so, remove the bay leaf, then serve.

MEDITERRANEAN-STYLE
Lamb Shanks

🕐 **15 MINS** | 🍲 **VARIABLE** (SEE BELOW) | 🔥 **582 CALS** PER SERVING

Slow-cooking – whether in the oven, pressure cooker or slow cooker – is a wonderful way to bring out the beautiful, rich and tender taste of lamb. The delicious ingredients in this recipe make it perfect for wowing at a dinner party, without the need for high-calorie ingredients. *(Pictured overleaf)*

Special Occasion

Use GF stock cubes

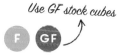

SERVES 4

4 lamb shanks (all visible fat removed) – about 14–16 oz each
sea salt and freshly ground black pepper
low-calorie cooking spray
1 tbsp Worcestershire sauce, plus a dash to deglaze
1 cup beef stock (1 beef stock cube dissolved in 1 cup boiling water)
1 large onion, roughly chopped
2 celery sticks, roughly chopped
2 medium carrots, roughly chopped
3 garlic cloves, smashed and peeled
2 tbsp tomato paste
1 (14 oz) tin chopped tomatoes
2 fresh tomatoes, chopped
1 beef stock cube (in addition to the one above)
1 tsp fish sauce
1 tbsp balsamic vinegar
1 tsp dried oregano
1 tsp dried rosemary
½ tsp dried thyme
generous handful of fresh parsley
cooked couscous, to serve (optional)

OVEN METHOD
🍲 2½–3 HOURS

Season the lamb with salt and pepper. Spray a large frying pan with low-calorie cooking spray and add the lamb shanks. Brown them over a medium heat for around 5 minutes until browned all over (this boosts the flavour).

Place the lamb in a large lidded casserole dish. Preheat the oven to 350°F (fan 325°F).

Deglaze the frying pan with a dash of the Worcestershire sauce and beef stock, scraping up any bits of meat stuck to the bottom of the pan – use a wooden spoon for this. Add the onion, celery, carrots and garlic. Fry for a few minutes, coating them in the deglaze mix, until the onion starts to colour, then add the tomato paste and fry for 3–5 minutes.

Pour the pan mixture into the dish on top of the lamb shanks. Add all the remaining ingredients (except the parsley), making sure to crumble in the stock cube. Cover and cook in the oven for 2–2½ hours until the lamb is tender, checking a few times during cooking to see if you need to add a little more liquid.

Remove the shanks from the dish and heat the sauce until it reaches the desired consistency (you may want to pass the liquid through a fat strainer as lamb is naturally quite fatty). Stir through the chopped parsley and serve with couscous, if desired, pouring the sauce over the top.

More methods overleaf …

MEDITERRANEAN-STYLE LAMB SHANKS ... *Continued*

ELECTRIC PRESSURE COOKER METHOD
🍲 50 MINS

Season the lamb with salt and pepper. Spray a large frying pan with low-calorie cooking spray and add the lamb shanks. Brown them over a medium heat for around 5 minutes until browned all over (this boosts the flavour).

Transfer the shanks to the pressure cooker.

Deglaze the frying pan with a dash of the Worcestershire sauce and beef stock, scraping up any bits of meat stuck to the bottom of the pan – use a wooden spoon for this. Add the onion, celery, carrots and garlic. Fry for a few minutes, coating them in the deglaze mix, until the onion starts to colour, then add the tomato paste and fry for 3–5 minutes.

Pour the contents of the pan into the pressure cooker, on top of the lamb shanks. Add all the remaining ingredients (except the parsley), making sure to crumble in the stock cube.

Pressure-cook on Manual/Stew setting for 45 minutes. Allow the pressure to release naturally (Natural Pressure Release/NPR).

Remove the lamb shanks from the pressure cooker and set it to Sauté/Browning to reduce the sauce until it reaches the desired consistency (you may want to pass the liquid through a fat strainer as lamb is naturally quite fatty).

Stir through the chopped parsley and serve with couscous, if desired, pouring the sauce over the top.

SLOW COOKER METHOD
🍲 4–8 HOURS

Season the lamb with salt and pepper. Spray a large frying pan with low-calorie cooking spray and add the lamb shanks. Brown them over a medium heat for around 5 minutes until browned all over (this boosts the flavour).

Transfer the shanks to the slow cooker.

Deglaze the frying pan with a dash of the Worcestershire sauce and beef stock, scraping up any bits of meat stuck to the bottom of the pan – use a wooden spoon for this. Add the onion, celery, carrots and garlic. Fry for a few minutes, coating them in the deglaze mix, until the onion starts to colour, then add the tomato paste and fry for 3–5 minutes.

Pour the contents of the pan into the slow cooker on top of the lamb shanks. Add all the remaining ingredients (except the parsley), making sure to crumble in the stock cube.

Cook on Medium for 4–5 hours or Low for 7–8 hours.

When the lamb is tender remove the shanks from the slow cooker. Cook the sauce uncovered on High for around 30 minutes or until it reaches the desired consistency (you may want to pass the liquid through a fat strainer as lamb is naturally quite fatty).

Stir through the chopped parsley and serve with couscous, if desired, pouring the sauce over the top.

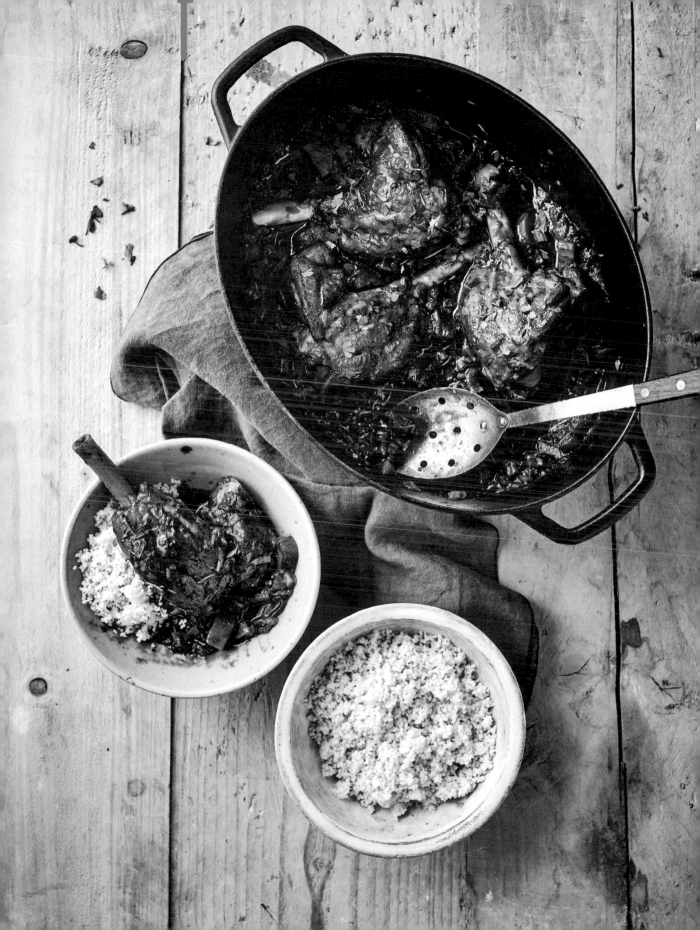

GOULASH

🕐 **15 MINS** | 🍲 **VARIABLE** (SEE BELOW) | 🔥 **357 CALS** PER SERVING

Rich with paprika and tomatoes, this goulash is simmered over a low heat for a long period of time – you can use the oven or a slow cooker with similar effect – and the meat becomes deliciously tender and releases its flavour into the sauce. Serve alongside our Easy Pilaf Rice with Chickpeas (page 209) and you're onto a winning, filling and super-tasty Hungarian feast!

───────── *Weekly Indulgence* ─────────

Use GF stock cubes ↘

SERVES 4

1 lb 2 oz stewing steak (all visible fat removed), cut into bite-sized pieces

3 tbsp smoked sweet paprika

low-calorie cooking spray

1 large onion, cut into large chunks

1 red pepper, deseeded and cut into large chunks

1 yellow pepper, deseeded and cut into large chunks

¾ tsp garlic granules

2 medium carrots, cut into 1 in chunks

6 oz medium potatoes, peeled and cut into 1 in chunks

2 tbsp tomato paste

1 (14 oz) tin chopped tomatoes

2 cups beef stock (2 beef stock pots such as Knorr concentrated beef stock, dissolved in 2 cups boiling water)

sea salt and freshly ground black pepper

steamed or pickled red cabbage, to serve (optional)

OVEN METHOD
🍲 2–2½ HOURS

Toss the steak in the paprika until well coated. Preheat the oven to 375°F (fan 350°F).

Spray a large casserole dish with low-calorie cooking spray and place over a medium heat, add the meat and cook for 5 minutes until browned. Remove and set aside.

Return the dish to a medium heat, spray with some more low-calorie cooking spray, then add the onion and peppers. Cook for 3–4 minutes until they start to soften, then return the browned meat to the pan and add the garlic granules, carrots, potatoes, tomato paste, chopped tomatoes and stock. Stir well and bring to the boil, then cover with a tight-fitting lid and cook in the oven for 1½–2 hours or until the meat is tender.

Taste, and season with salt and pepper if necessary. Serve with red cabbage, if you like.

More methods overleaf ...

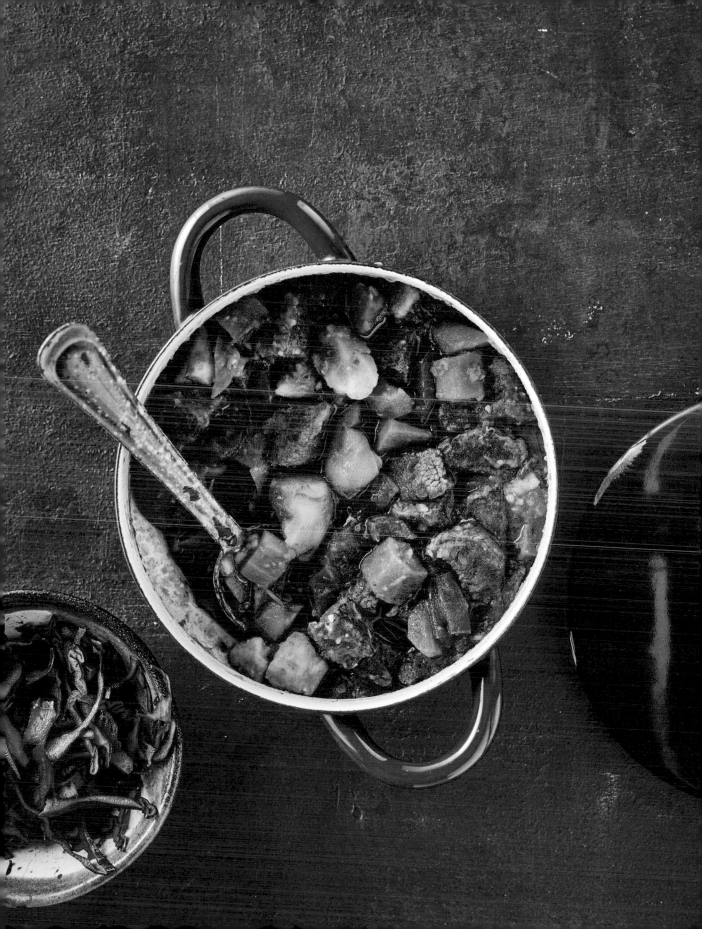

GOULASH *... Continued*

ELECTRIC PRESSURE COOKER METHOD
🍲 **45 MINS**

Toss the steak in the paprika until well coated.

Set the pressure cooker to Sauté/Browning, then spray with low-calorie cooking spray. Add the meat and sauté for about 5 minutes until browned. Set aside.

Add a little more low-calorie cooking spray to the pressure cooker and sauté the onions for 3–4 minutes until they start to soften.

Add the meat, peppers, garlic granules, carrots, potatoes, tomato paste, tomatoes and stock to the pressure cooker.

Pressure-cook on Manual/Stew setting for 30 minutes. Allow the pressure to release naturally (Natural Pressure Release/NPR).
If the sauce is a little thin you can remove the lid and cook on Sauté/Browning for a few minutes to reduce the liquid.

Taste, and season with salt and pepper if necessary.

Serve with red cabbage, if you like.

SLOW COOKER METHOD
🍲 **4½–7 HOURS**

Toss the steak in the paprika until well coated.

Spray a frying pan with low-calorie cooking spray and place over a medium heat. Add the meat and cook for 5 minutes until browned on all sides.

Place the browned meat in the slow cooker with the onion, peppers, garlic granules, carrots and potatoes. Add the tomato paste to the slow cooker, along with the tomatoes and stock. Stir well, set the slow cooker to High, cover and cook for 4½ hours, or on Low for 6–7 hours until the meat and veg are tender.

Taste, and season with salt and pepper if necessary.

Serve with red cabbage, if you like.

BEEF *in* RED WINE
with SHALLOTS

🕐 **15 MINS** | 🍲 **VARIABLE** (SEE BELOW) | 💧 **332 CALS** PER SERVING

Using red or white wine stock pots in dishes is an easy way to reduce the calories without compromising on the taste. They're just perfect for dishes like this tender slow-cooked beef with sweet shallots, combined with some classic root vegetables. Classically French in style, this meal will feel like such a treat on a cold evening. *(Pictured overleaf)*

Weekly Indulgence

Use GF stock cubes

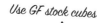

F **GF**

SERVES 4

4 good-sized stewing steaks
  (all visible fat removed), left
  whole – around 4½ oz each
sea salt and freshly ground
  black pepper
low-calorie cooking spray
8 large shallots, cut lengthways
2 sprigs of thyme
mashed potato, to serve (optional)

FOR THE GRAVY
½ onion, roughly chopped
1 small carrot, roughly chopped
1 cup peeled and roughly chopped
  rutabaga
1 small potato, peeled and
  roughly chopped
2½ cups water
2 red wine stock pot
1 beef stock pot (such as Knorr
  concentrated beef stock)

OVEN METHOD
🍲 **3½–4 HOURS**

To make the gravy, put the onion, carrot, rutabaga and potato in a saucepan with the water, bring to the boil, then turn the heat down to low and simmer for 30 minutes, until the vegetables are soft. Add the wine and the stock pot, remove from the heat and blend with a stick blender until smooth.

Season the meat well with salt and pepper.

Preheat the oven to 350°F (fan 325°F).

Spray a large frying pan with low-calorie cooking spray and place over a medium–high heat. Add the steaks to the pan and brown on both sides, then place them in a casserole dish. (If you have a small frying pan you may need to do this in batches to avoid overcrowding the pan.)

Scatter the shallots over the steaks and pour over the gravy. Place the thyme on top, cover and cook in the oven for 3–3½ hours.

Check the meat is tender after 3–3½ hours, and return to the oven for another 30 minutes if necessary. Serve as it is, or with mashed potato.

More methods overleaf…

ELECTRIC PRESSURE COOKER METHOD
50 MINS

To make the gravy, put the onion, carrot, rutabaga and potato in a saucepan with the water, bring to the boil, then turn the heat down to low and simmer for 30 minutes, until the vegetables are soft. Add the wine and the stock pot, remove from the heat and blend with a stick blender until smooth.

Season the meat well with salt and pepper.

Spray a frying pan with cooking spray and place over a medium–high heat. Add the steaks to the pan and brown on both sides, then transfer to the pressure cooker. (If you have a small frying pan you may need to do this in batches to avoid overcrowding the pan.)

Brown the shallots in the same pan you used for browning the steaks, then scatter them over the steaks in the pressure cooker.

Pour over the gravy and add another ¾ cup water. Place the thyme on top.

Put the lid on and set the pressure cooker to Manual/Stew and pressure-cook for 40 minutes. Allow the pressure to release naturally (Natural Pressure Release/NPR).

When the pressure has released, check the meat is tender and serve. If the sauce is a bit thick just add a little water. If it's too thin set the pressure cooker to Sauté/Browning and allow it to reduce slightly. Serve as it is, or with mashed potato.

SLOW COOKER METHOD
4–9 HOURS

To make the gravy, put the onion, carrot, rutabaga and potato in a saucepan with the water, bring to the boil, then turn the heat down to low and simmer for 30 minutes, until the vegetables are soft. Add the wine and the stock pot, remove from the heat and blend with a stick blender until smooth.

Season the meat well with salt and pepper.

Spray a frying pan with cooking spray and place over a medium–high heat. Add the steaks to the pan and brown on both sides, then transfer to the slow cooker. (If you have a small frying pan you may need to do this in batches to avoid overcrowding the pan.)

Scatter the shallots over the steaks.

Pour over the gravy and pour in another ¾ cup water. Place the thyme on top. Cover, and cook on High for 4–6 hours, or on Low for 8–9 hours.

Check the meat and if it's not tender, continue cooking for another hour or so. Serve as it is, or with mashed potato.

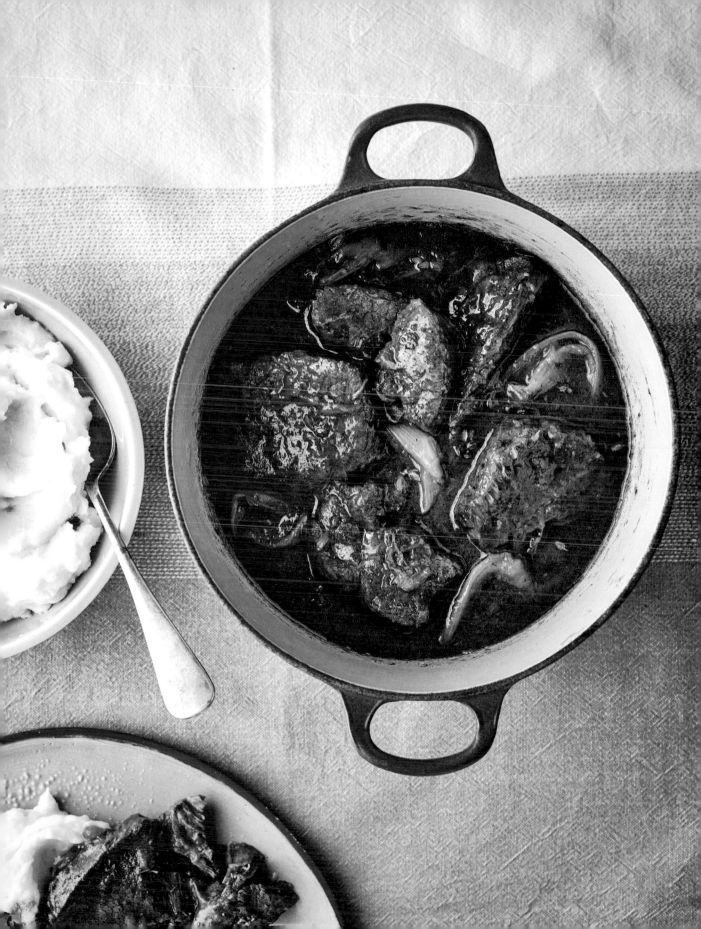

POULET *au* VINAIGRE

🕐 **15 MINS** | 🍲 **30 MINS** | 🔥 **197 CALS** PER SERVING

This classic, creamy French dish usually uses ingredients only the French can get away with! Half a bottle of sherry, anyone? Luckily, with some clever ingredients – a white wine stock pot and some white wine vinegar – you can re-create the lovely sharpness of the original dish, while backing down on some of those calories. You can imagine you're in a *gîte* in the South of France while it bubbles away!

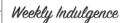

Weekly Indulgence

Use GF stock cubes

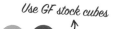

F **GF**

SERVES 4

low-calorie cooking spray
8 chicken thighs (skin and visible
  fat removed)
½ onion, finely chopped
2 garlic cloves, crushed
2 tomatoes, peeled, deseeded
  and diced
1 tsp tomato paste
½ tsp English mustard powder
1¼ cups chicken stock (1 chicken
  stock cube dissolved in 1¼ cups
  boiling water)
1 white wine stock pot
3 tbsp white wine vinegar
5 tbsp low-fat cream cheese
1 tsp chopped fresh tarragon
steamed greens, to serve (optional)

Spray a large heavy-based pan (with a lid) with low-calorie cooking spray and place over a high heat. Add the chicken thighs and brown for 2–3 minutes each side, then remove from the pan and set aside.

Reduce the heat, spray with a little more low-calorie cooking spray, then add the onion and garlic and cook for 3 minutes, or until slightly softened but not coloured. Add the diced tomatoes, tomato paste and mustard powder and cook for 1 minute.

Pour in the stock, stock pot and white wine vinegar, then stir well and bring to a simmer. Return the chicken pieces to the pan, cover with a lid, and cook over a low heat for 20–25 minutes, until the chicken is cooked through. The juices should run clear when you pierce the thighs with a sharp knife.

Remove the chicken from the pan and cover with foil to keep warm.

Turn the heat up and bring the sauce to a rapid boil for 6–8 minutes, or until the sauce starts to thicken (it should be the consistency of light cream). Stir in the cream cheese and chopped tarragon, then return the chicken to the pan to warm through.

Serve with steamed greens and/or mashed potato, if desired.

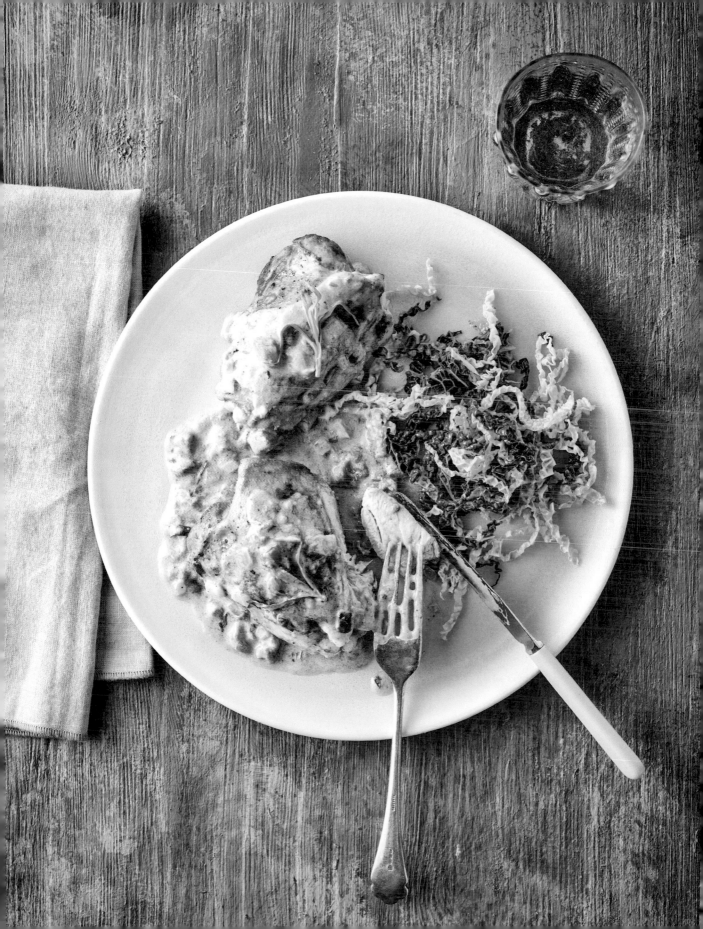

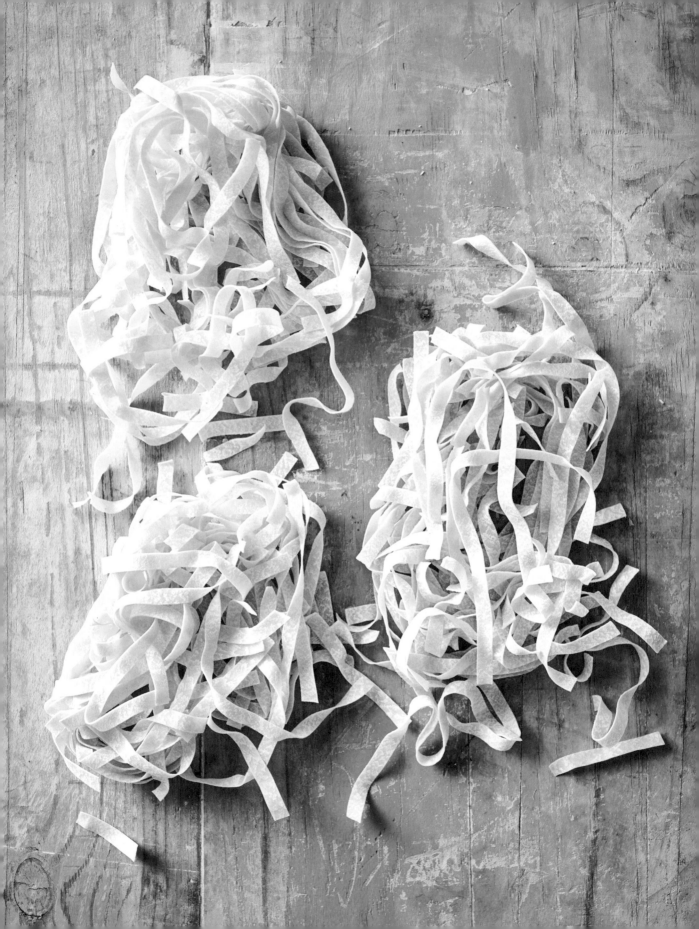

The Cock and Bull is

ABSOLUTELY AMAZING

could have been the

REAL THING

GILLIAN

"

MEDITERRANEAN-STYLE LAMB SHANKS, wow, so full of *flavour*. Definitely making these again.

JULIE

Wow wow wow – the **LAMB GUVECH** was a big hit in my household.

CLAIRE

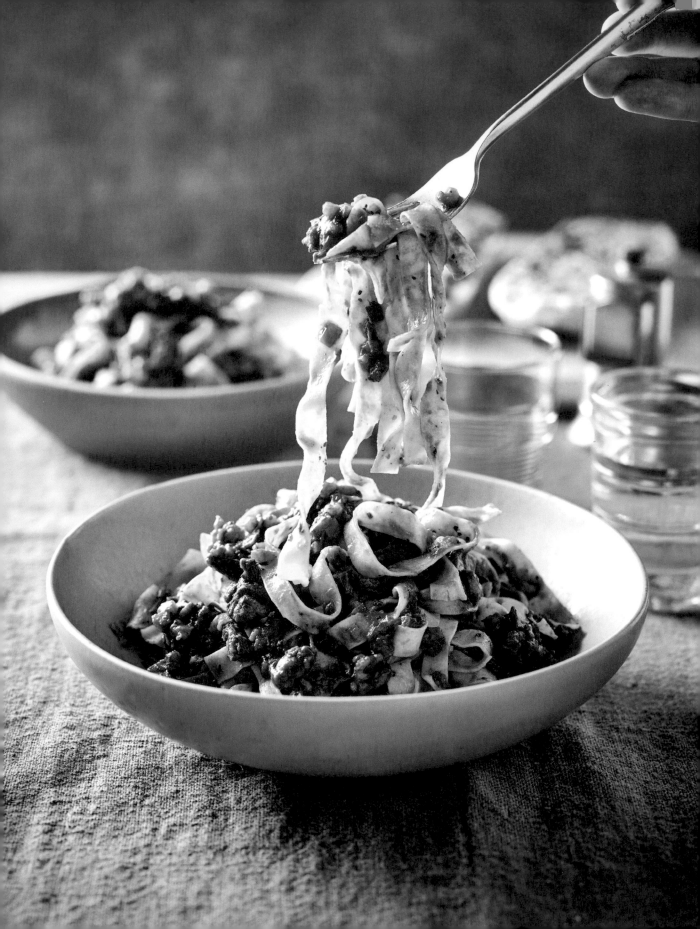

BEEF RAGU
Fettuccine

🕐 **10 MINS** | 🍲 **VARIABLE** (SEE BELOW) | 🔥 **445 CALS** PER SERVING

This fettuccine dish is a great family meal. Rich with beef and tomatoes, it makes the perfect end to a long day. Serve with a small glass of red wine and side salad for a really indulgent meal, or just on its own as the family descends for dinnertime en masse!

─────────────── *Everyday Light* ───────────────

F

SERVES 4

10½ oz stewing steak (all visible
    fat removed), cut into
    bite-sized chunks
sea salt and freshly ground
    black pepper
low-calorie cooking spray
1 onion, finely diced
1 medium carrot, finely diced
1 zucchini, finely diced
1½ cups thinly sliced mushrooms
2 garlic cloves, crushed
1 (500g) carton passata (tomato
    puree; about 2 cups)
1¼ cups beef stock (2 beef
    stock cubes dissolved in
    1¼ cups boiling water)
2 tsp dried oregano
2 tsp dried basil
1 tsp Worcestershire sauce
2 tbsp tomato paste
¼ cup pearl barley
7 oz dried fettuccine
grated Parmesan, to serve (optional)

STOVETOP METHOD
🍲 **2 HOURS 30 MINS**

Season the meat well with salt and pepper.

Spray a large saucepan with low-calorie cooking spray. On a high heat, fry off the meat for about 10 minutes until browned.

When the meat is browned, add the veg and sauté for another couple of minutes. Add all the remaining ingredients apart from the pearl barley and pasta. Mix well, pop a lid on the saucepan and simmer on a low heat for 1 hour, stirring occasionally.

After an hour, add the pearl barley to the ragu and stir. Put the lid back on and cook for a further hour until the beef is very tender.

Around 20 minutes before the ragu has finished cooking, put on a pan of water and cook the pasta according to the instructions on the packet.

Add the cooked, drained pasta to the ragu, combine, and serve, topped with grated Parmesan (remember to count the calories if using it!).

More methods overleaf …

ELECTRIC PRESSURE COOKER METHOD
🍲 **30 MINS**

Season the meat well with salt and pepper.

Place a large pan of water onto the stovetop to boil for the pasta.

Set the pressure cooker to Sauté/Browning setting and spray it with a little low-calorie cooking spray. Brown the meat in the pressure cooker in small batches for a few minutes then set aside.

Add the vegetables and garlic to the pressure cooker and sauté for 2 minutes, then press the Off button and add the remaining ingredients, including the browned meat (but not the pasta and Parmesan), to the cooker. Close the lid, set to Manual/Stew setting and pressure-cook for 30 minutes, ensuring that the venting valve is closed.

Cook the pasta in the boiling water according to the packet instructions, then drain.

When the pressure cooker has finished cooking, use the Quick Pressure Release method and stir the cooked pasta into the ragu.

Serve immediately, with a sprinkle of Parmesan (remember to count the calories if using it!).

SLOW COOKER METHOD
🍲 **6 HOURS**

Season the meat well with salt and pepper.

Spray a large frying pan with a little low-calorie cooking spray, then place over a medium heat, add the meat and sauté for a few minutes until browned. Once browned, add the veg and garlic and sauté for a further 2 minutes.

Tip the contents of the pan into the slow cooker then add all the remaining ingredients, except the pasta and Parmesan. Set the slow cooker to Medium-high and cook for 5–6 hours or until the meat starts to break up.

Place a large pan of water onto the stovetop to boil for the pasta. Cook the pasta according to the packet instructions, then drain and stir into the ragu.

Serve immediately, with a sprinkle of Parmesan (remember to count the calories if using it!).

LAMB GUVECH

⏱ 10 MINS | **🍲 VARIABLE** (SEE BELOW) | **🔥 356 CALS** PER SERVING

Lamb is typically a fatty meat, so it's often avoided in lower-calorie recipes. However, when cooked slowly like it is in this dish, with its fat trimmed off, the meat is still deliciously tender. While heavy on prep, this Bulgarian dish packs a real flavour punch and is worth the initial effort. You can leave it slowly cooking while you get on with other things. *(Pictured overleaf)*

Weekly Indulgence

Use GF stock cubes
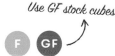

SERVES 4

1 lb 2 oz lamb (all visible fat
   removed), diced
sea salt and freshly ground
   black pepper
low-calorie cooking spray
   (except if cooking in the
   slow cooker)
1 onion, diced
4 garlic cloves, finely chopped
1 green pepper, deseeded and diced
1 red pepper, deseeded and diced
10 mushrooms, sliced
2 lamb stock cubes
1 beef stock cube
2 bay leaves
2 tsp chopped fresh parsley
generous pinch of dried chile flakes
2 (14 oz) tins chopped tomatoes
1 tsp smoked sweet paprika
1 tsp ground cumin
1 tsp red wine vinegar
1 tbsp tomato paste
Easy Pilaf Rice with Chickpeas
   (see page 209), to serve

OVEN METHOD
🍲 1 HOUR 40 MINS

Season the lamb with salt and pepper.

Preheat the oven to 350°F (fan 325°F).

Spray a large ovenproof casserole dish with low-calorie cooking spray. Add the lamb to the dish and brown the diced lamb for around 5 minutes over a medium heat. Set aside.

Add some more low-calorie cooking spray and sauté the onion and garlic for 3–4 minutes over a medium heat, until they start to soften. Return the lamb to the pot, along with 1 cup water.

Add all the remaining ingredients. Stir well, cover with the lid and cook for 1½ hours. Check after 1 hour to make sure that the liquid hasn't evaporated. If it has, add some more water.

After the full cooking time, check the meat is cooked. If not, continue cooking for another 30 minutes.

When the meat is cooked, check the seasoning and add some more salt and pepper if necessary. If the Guvech needs thickening return to the oven without the lid and allow it to reduce slightly. Serve with Easy Pilaf Rice with Chickpeas (see page 209).

More methods overleaf …

ELECTRIC PRESSURE COOKER METHOD
🍲 1 HOUR

Season the lamb with salt and pepper.

Set the pressure cooker to Sauté/Browning, spray with some low-calorie cooking spray, then brown the diced lamb for around 5 minutes and set aside.

Add some more low-calorie cooking spray and sauté the onion and garlic for 3–4 minutes, until they start to soften. Return the lamb to the pressure cooker, along with 1 cup water.

Add all the remaining ingredients. Set the pressure cooker to Manual/Stew and pressure-cook for 50 minutes. Allow the pressure to release naturally (Natural Pressure Release/NPR).

If the Guvech needs thickening remove the lid and set the pressure cooker to Sauté/Browning for 5 minutes until the sauce has reduced slightly.

Taste, and add some more salt and pepper if necessary. Serve with Easy Pilaf Rice with Chickpeas (see page 209).

SLOW COOKER METHOD
🍲 5–8 HOURS

Season the lamb with salt and pepper.

Put all of the ingredients, apart from salt and pepper, in the slow cooker. Stir well, set the slow cooker to High, cover and cook for 5 hours, or on Low for 8 hours, until the meat and vegetables are tender.

Taste, and season with salt and pepper if necessary. Serve with Easy Pilaf Rice with Chickpeas (see page 209).

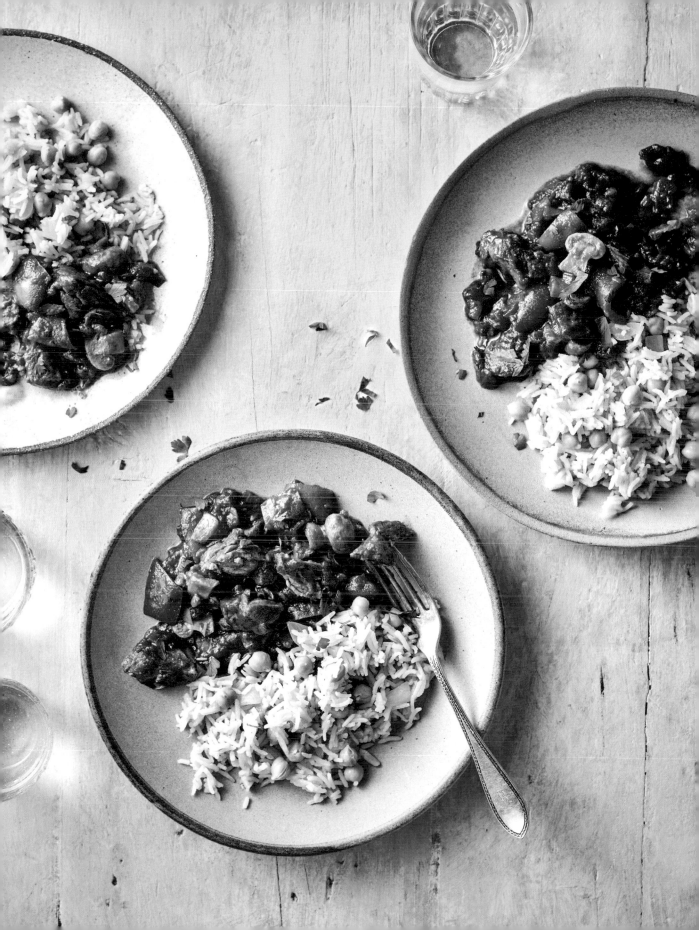

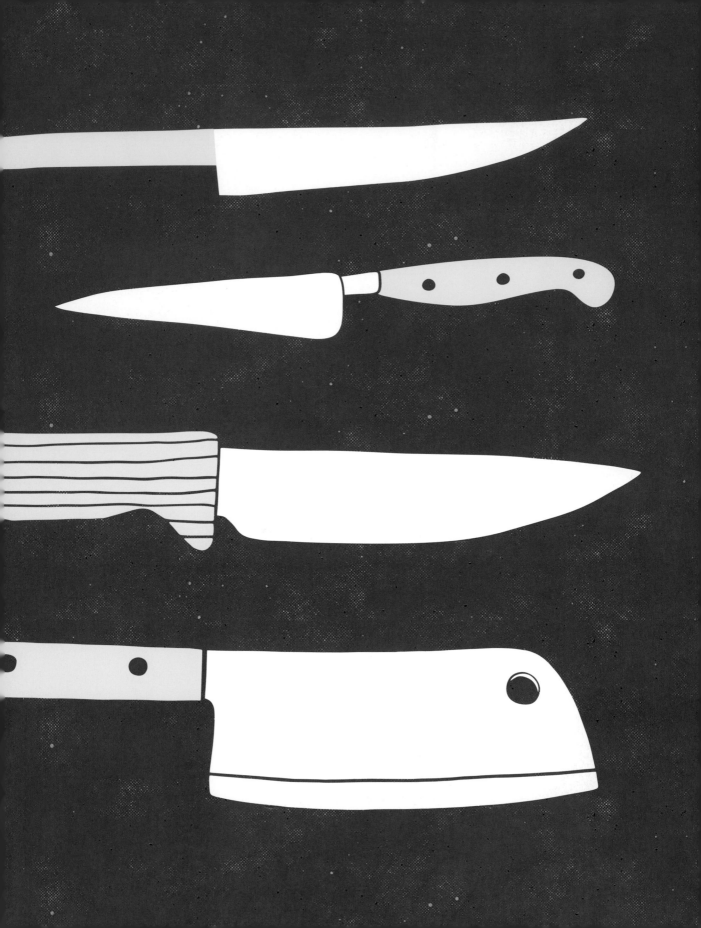

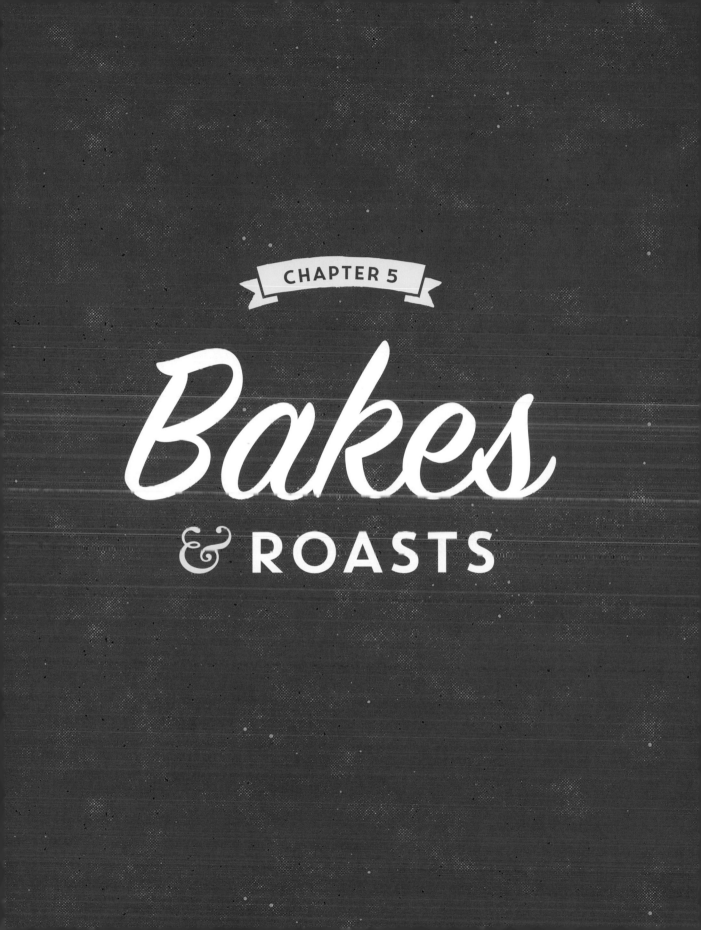

CHAPTER 5

Bakes
& ROASTS

BACON *and* CHEESE
POTATO SKINS

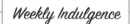 10 MINS | 🍲 40 MINS | 🔥 263 CALS PER SERVING

When you think of loaded potato skins, it's easy to assume they're laden with The Bad Things. With a few simple substitutes, however, you can re-create all the flavour so they feel like a cheesy, indulgent treat, without all the calories.

Weekly Indulgence

SERVES 4

4 medium potatoes
6 Canadian bacon medallions
5 scallions, trimmed and
    thinly sliced
scant 1 cup fat-free cottage cheese
sea salt and freshly ground
    black pepper
⅓ cup grated Parmesan

Scrub the potatoes, pierce them with the prongs of a fork and microwave them until they are cooked. (If you don't have a microwave, preheat the oven to 400°F [fan 375°F] and bake the potatoes for 1¼–1½ hours until golden brown and cooked through.)

Cook the bacon medallions under the broiler, in the oven or in a dry frying pan on the stovetop, then set aside.

Preheat the oven to 400°F (fan 375°F).

Allow the cooked potatoes to cool slightly (just enough so you can handle them without burning yourself) then cut them in half lengthways and scoop out the potato into a bowl.

Chop the bacon into small pieces.

Mash the potato roughly with a fork, then stir in the scallions and cottage cheese. Season with salt and pepper to taste.

Spoon the mixture back into the empty potato shells, pressing it in slightly. Top each potato with the chopped bacon and an even sprinkle of Parmesan. Place the filled potato shells on a baking tray and cook in the oven for about 20 minutes, or until the Parmesan is melted and golden brown, and serve.

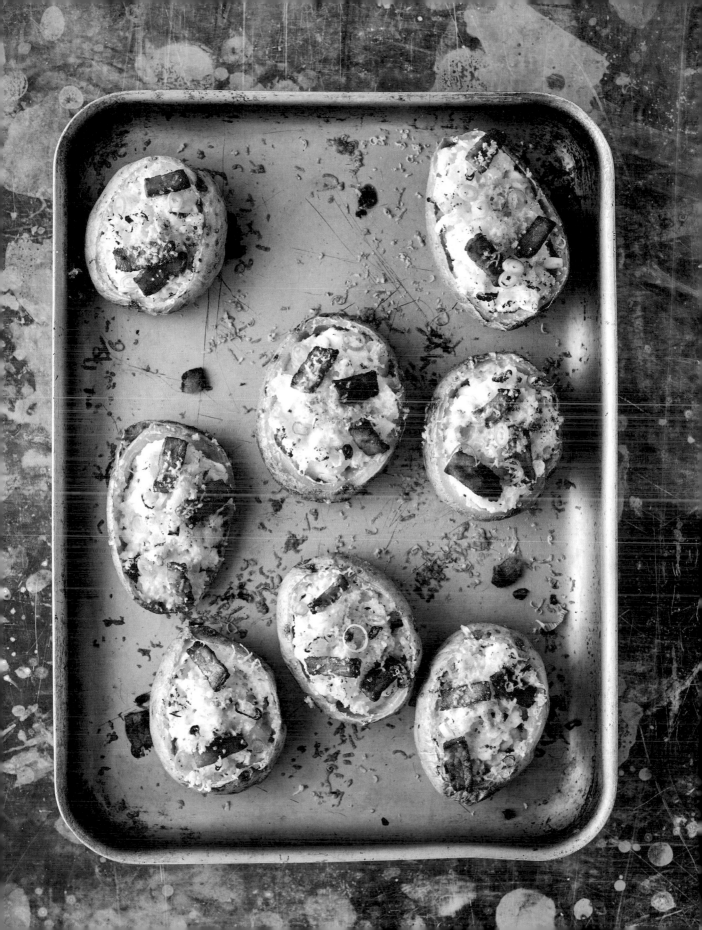

Hunter's CHICKEN

🕐 **10 MINS** | 🍲 **VARIABLE** (SEE BELOW) | 🔥 **343 CALS** PER SERVING

A British pub classic, this hunter's chicken is ideal for family meals and dinner parties alike. With some reduced-fat cheese grilled and crisped up on top, it really feels like a rich, indulgent treat. We have included recipes for using a slow cooker or cooking in the oven. You'll want to open your own pub just to serve it!

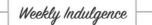

Weekly Indulgence

SERVES 4

4 chicken breasts (skin and visible fat removed)
4 Canadian bacon medallions
½ onion, diced
2 garlic cloves, crushed
1 (14 oz) tin chopped tomatoes
1 tbsp tomato paste
juice of ½ lemon
1 tbsp BBQ seasoning
¼ tsp sweet smoked paprika (or chile powder or plain paprika if you don't have this)
1 tbsp balsamic vinegar
2 tbsp Worcestershire sauce
2 tbsp white wine vinegar
1 tbsp hot sauce
1 tsp mustard powder
1 tsp granulated sweetener
⅔ cup grated reduced-fat Cheddar

OVEN METHOD
🍲 **1 HOUR**

Preheat the oven to 350°F (fan 325°F). Wrap a bacon medallion around the middle of each chicken breast and secure it with a cocktail stick.

Put all of the remaining ingredients (except the cheese) in an ovenproof casserole dish with a tight-fitting lid. Place the chicken on top, cover with the lid and cook in the oven for 1 hour. When the time is up, check that the chicken is cooked. Remove it from the dish and set aside. Blitz the sauce in the casserole with a stick blender until smooth.

Place the cooked chicken in an ovenproof dish and remove the cocktail sticks. Pour the sauce over the chicken breasts and scatter over the cheese, dividing it equally among all four chicken breasts. Place under a hot broiler until the cheese is melted and has a nice golden colour.

SLOW COOKER METHOD
🍲 **2½–3 HOURS**

Wrap a bacon medallion around the middle of each chicken breast and secure it with a cocktail stick.

Put all the remaining ingredients (except the cheese) in the slow cooker and stir well. Place the wrapped chicken on top and put the lid on. Set to cook on High for 2½–3 hours. (Or set it to Low if you're leaving it on all day.)

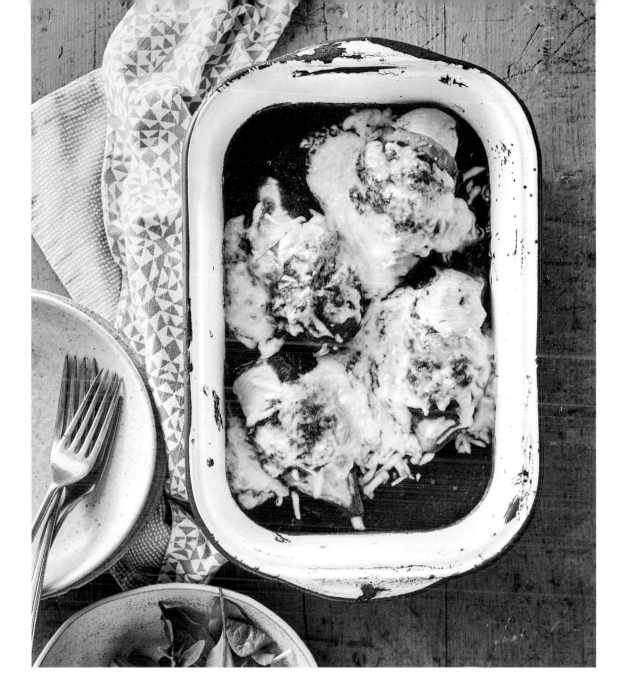

When the time is up, check that the chicken is cooked. Remove it from the slow cooker and set aside. Blitz the remaining sauce in the slow cooker pot with a stick blender until smooth.

Place the cooked chicken in an ovenproof dish and remove the cocktail sticks. Pour the sauce over the chicken breasts and scatter over the cheese, dividing it equally among all four chicken breasts. Place under a hot broiler until the cheese is melted and has a nice golden colour.

BACON, ONION *and* POTATO BAKE

🕐 **10 MINS** | 🍲 **1 HOUR 15 MINS** | 🔥 **415 CALS** PER SERVING

This bake is one of Kay's childhood favourites, when it was affectionately known as "Tin of Praters." It's one of those dishes that is ridiculously easy to make and uses minimal ingredients and yet … the taste! Seriously! We predict this will become an absolute family hit.

Weekly Indulgence

Use a GF stock cube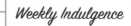

SERVES 4

2 onions, thinly sliced

2¼ lb medium potatoes, peeled and thinly sliced

16 Canadian bacon medallions (use more bacon if you wish, depending on pack size, but this will affect cals count)

scant 1 cup chicken or vegetable stock (1 chicken or vegetable stock cube dissolved in scant 1 c boiling water)

sea salt and freshly ground black pepper

⅓ cup grated reduced-fat Cheddar

Preheat the oven to 400°F (fan 375°F).

Spread a layer of sliced onion on the bottom of an ovenproof dish. Arrange a layer of sliced potato and bacon on top of the onions, alternating a couple of slices of potato with a piece of bacon. Next, add another layer of onions. Repeat until you have used up all the bacon and potatoes. You should have at least three layers.

Pour the stock over the top, then season with a little salt and pepper. Cover with foil and seal the foil tightly around the dish.

Cook in the oven for 1 hour, then remove the foil and check that the potato is cooked. If it's not, re-cover and return it to the oven for a bit longer. When it is cooked, sprinkle the cheese over the top, then return to the oven for another 10–15 minutes, or until the cheese has melted and is golden brown.

Tip
Use floury potatoes like Idaho or russet, as they absorb a lot of liquid and flavour.

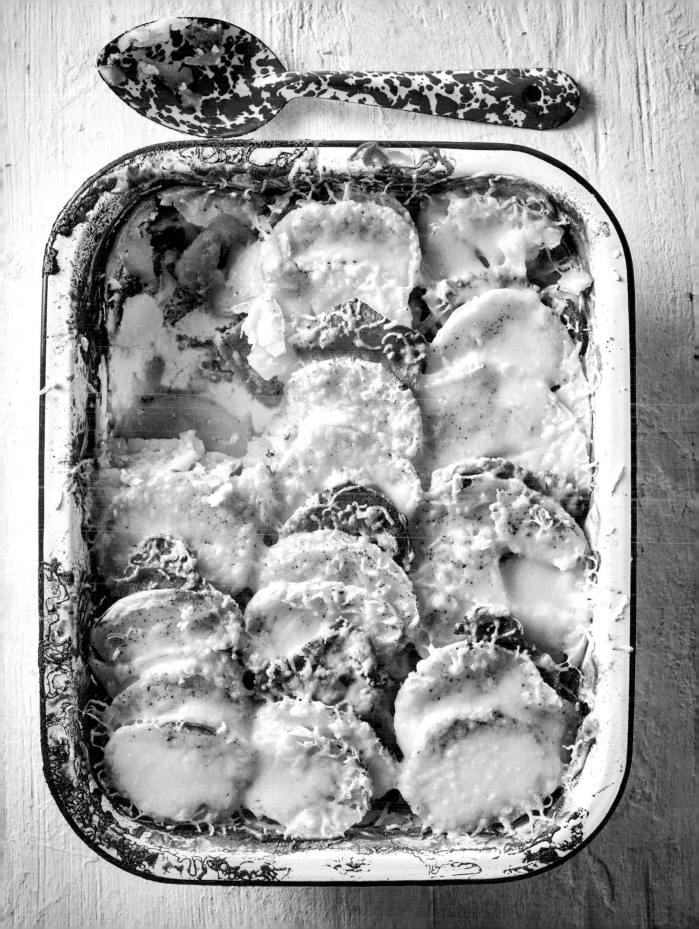

BUFFALO
SKINS

🕐 **5 MINS** | 🍲 **30 MINS** | 🔥 **161 CALS** PER SERVING

Swapping out white potatoes for sweet potatoes is an instant way to reduce calorie intake. Balancing the taste of sweet potato with some classic buffalo hot sauce and some golden, melted cheese, these are the perfect healthy, go-to indulgence.

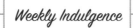

Weekly Indulgence

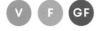

SERVES 4

4 medium sweet potatoes
5 scallions, trimmed and
 chopped
3 tbsp grated reduced-fat Cheddar
5 tbsp low-fat cream cheese
1 tsp buffalo wings hot sauce
sea salt and freshly ground
 black pepper
3 tbsp grated Parmesan (or
 vegetarian hard cheese)
green salad, to serve

Pierce the skins of the sweet potatoes and microwave them for around 10 minutes or until they are cooked, then leave them to cool slightly. (If you don't have a microwave, preheat the oven to 400°F [fan 375°F] and bake the potatoes for 35–45 minutes until cooked through.)

Preheat the oven to 400°F (fan 375°F).

Cut the cooked sweet potatoes in half lengthways, then scoop out the inside of each half and place it in a bowl. Mash it roughly with a fork, then stir in the scallions, Cheddar, cream cheese and hot sauce. Season to taste with salt and pepper. (You can freeze the filled sweet potatoes at this point for cooking on another day.)

Place the empty sweet potato shells on a baking tray. Spoon the mixture back into the empty shells, pressing it in slightly. Sprinkle the Parmesan evenly over the top of each potato and cook in the oven for about 20 minutes, or until the cheese is melted and golden brown. Serve warm or at room temperature with a fresh green salad.

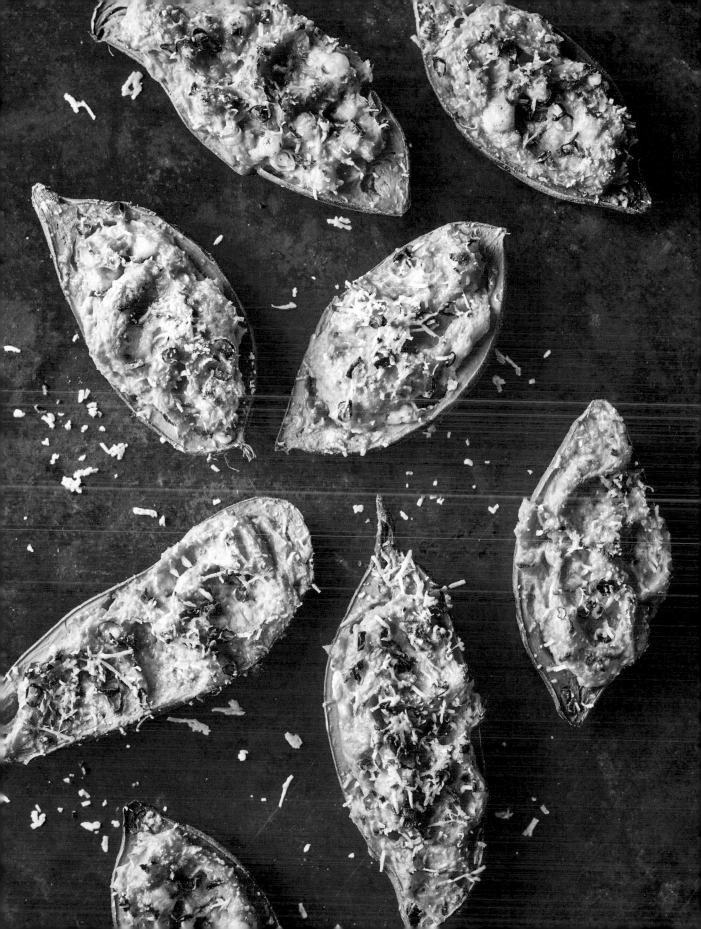

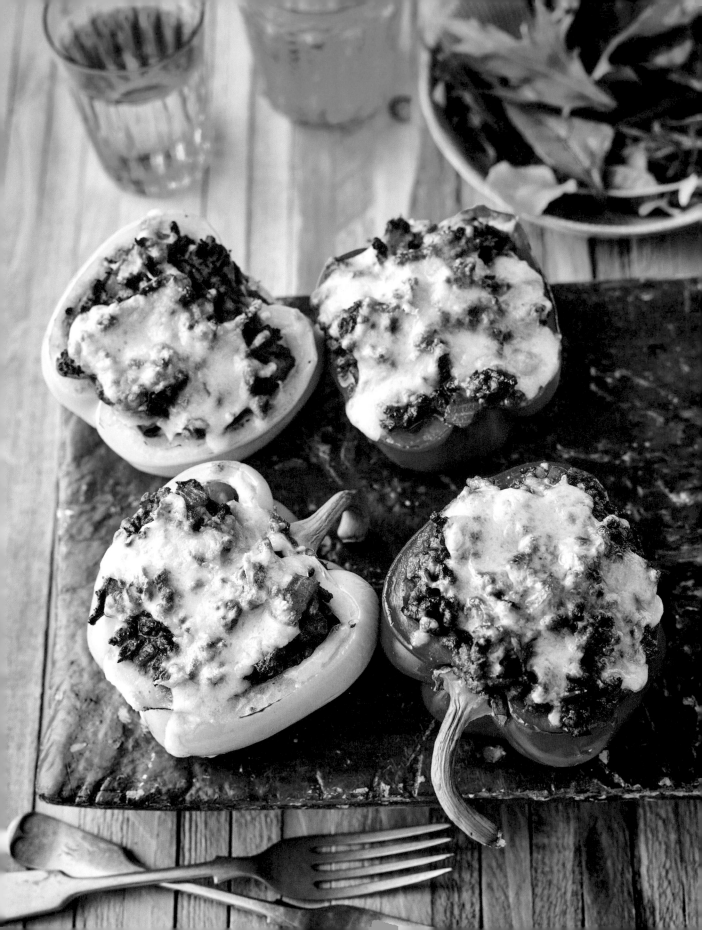

SLOPPY JOES

🕐 **10 MINS** | 🍲 **25 MINS** | 🔥 **268 CALS** PER SERVING

Sloppy Joes are a tasty, filling meat dish, typically served in a bun. Swapping the bun for some bell peppers and opting for lean ground beef makes this a much healthier version, but one that maintains the all-important delicious flavours of the original dish.

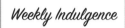

Weekly Indulgence

SERVES 4

low-calorie cooking spray
1 onion, finely diced
2 garlic cloves, finely chopped
1 green pepper, deseeded
    and finely diced
14 oz 5%-fat ground beef
1 tsp mustard powder
3 tbsp Worcestershire sauce
3 tbsp tomato paste
1 tbsp red wine vinegar
½ cup water
sea salt and freshly ground
    black pepper
1 red pepper, halved lengthways
    and deseeded
1 yellow pepper, halved lengthways
    and deseeded
⅓ cup grated reduced-fat Cheddar

Preheat the oven to 400°F (fan 375°F).

Spray a large frying pan with some low-calorie cooking spray and place over a medium heat. Add the onion, garlic and diced green pepper and cook for 4–5 minutes until they start to soften.

Add the ground beef, turn the heat up to high and cook for 5 minutes, stirring continuously and breaking it up with a wooden spoon.

Add the mustard powder, Worcestershire sauce, tomato paste, vinegar and water, turn the heat down to low and cook for another 3–4 minutes. Season to taste with salt and pepper.

Divide the beef mixture evenly among the four pepper halves. Scatter the cheese evenly over each pepper and place on a baking tray in the oven for 10 minutes, until the cheese is golden brown and the peppers are just cooked, but still have a bit of a crunch.

PORK *on* BALSAMIC LENTILS

⏱ **5 MINS** | 🍲 **30 MINS** | 🔥 **250 CALS** PER SERVING

Beans and pulses are some of the most satisfying and low-calorie ingredients you can cook with. Rich in protein and fibre, while having fantastic filling power, they can make tasty bases for hearty meals. If dried puy lentils are not available, use a 9 oz pack of ready-cooked lentils instead, and add them to the saucepan at the same time as you would add the cooked lentils.

--- *Everyday Light* ---

Use a GF stock cube

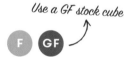

SERVES 4

1 lb 2 oz pork fillet (all visible fat removed), scored 4 times
12 sprigs of thyme
sea salt and freshly ground black pepper
scant ⅔ cup puy lentils, rinsed
low-calorie cooking spray
1 onion, finely chopped
2 medium carrots, cut into small dice
2 garlic cloves, crushed
⅔ cup chicken stock (1 chicken stock cube dissolved in ⅔ c boiling water)
1 (14 oz) tin chopped tomatoes
2 tbsp balsamic vinegar

Preheat the oven to 375°F (fan 350°F).

Stuff each cut in the pork fillet with a sprig of thyme and season well with salt and pepper. Place on a baking sheet and cook in the oven for 30 minutes.

Put the lentils in a saucepan, cover with three times the volume of water, bring to the boil and simmer gently for 20 minutes.

While the lentils are cooking, spray a large saucepan with low-calorie cooking spray and place over a low heat. Add the onion, carrots and crushed garlic and sauté for 10 minutes, or until the onions have softened. Strip the remaining thyme leaves from their sprigs and add the leaves to the pan, along with the stock and chopped tomatoes. Bring to a simmer and cook for 10 minutes.

Drain the lentils and add them to the pan. Stir in the balsamic vinegar and simmer for another 5 minutes.

Remove the pork from the oven, check it's cooked and cut it into twelve slices. Spoon the lentils onto four plates, top with the pork slices and serve.

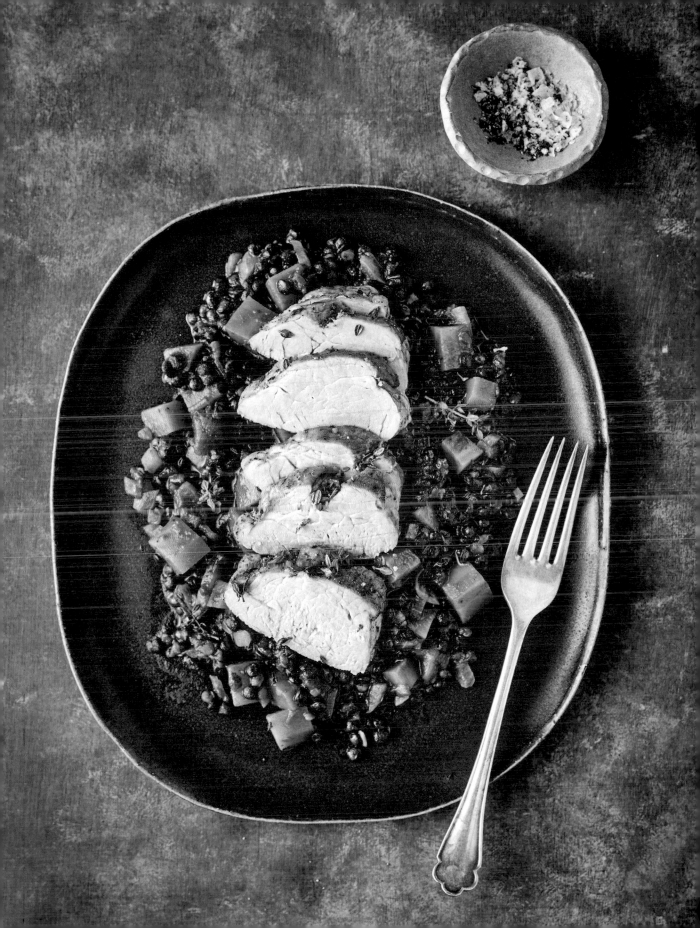

Yorkshire
PUDDING WRAP

🕐 **10 MINS** | 🍲 **10 MINS** | 🔥 **281 CALS** PER SERVING

We were working on a recipe for a giant Yorkshire pudding (see tip below) when we had an idea, which may or may not have been as a result of a carb craving. What if we made the batter work as a wrap for sandwich fillings? And thus the idea was born. We've perfected the recipe and it's now a Pinch of Nom favourite. Pack with lettuce leaves and roast beef slices for the perfect roast beef Yorkshire pudding wrap.

Weekly Indulgence

SERVES 2

low-calorie cooking spray
¼ cup all-purpose flour
2 medium eggs
⅓ cup skim milk
sea salt
6 mushrooms, sliced
½ onion, sliced
handful of arugula
2 slices of roast beef (trimmed of fat)
green salad, to serve

Preheat the oven to 450°F (fan 425°F) and spray a 9 in round cake tin generously with low-calorie cooking spray. Place the greased tin in the oven for 1–2 minutes until the oil starts foaming slightly.

Meanwhile, put the flour, eggs, milk and a pinch of salt in a decent-sized bowl and whisk by hand until the mixture is smooth.

Remove the hot tin from the oven, pour the batter in and return the tin to the oven for 8–10 minutes, or until the Yorkshire pudding has risen around the edges and is golden. You don't want it to be too crispy as this may make it more difficult to roll.

While the Yorkshire pudding is cooking, spray a frying pan with some low-calorie cooking spray and place it over a medium heat. Add the sliced mushrooms and onion and sauté for 4–5 minutes until they are browned and cooked.

Remove the Yorkshire pudding from the oven, remove it from the tin and cover it with the arugula. Add the beef slices and cooked onion and mushrooms, roll it up, slice it in half and serve with salad.

Tip
This batter also makes a fantastic Giant Yorkshire Pudding recipe – simply cook for a little longer in the oven (10–12 minutes) until the pudding has risen, is golden brown and holds its shape.

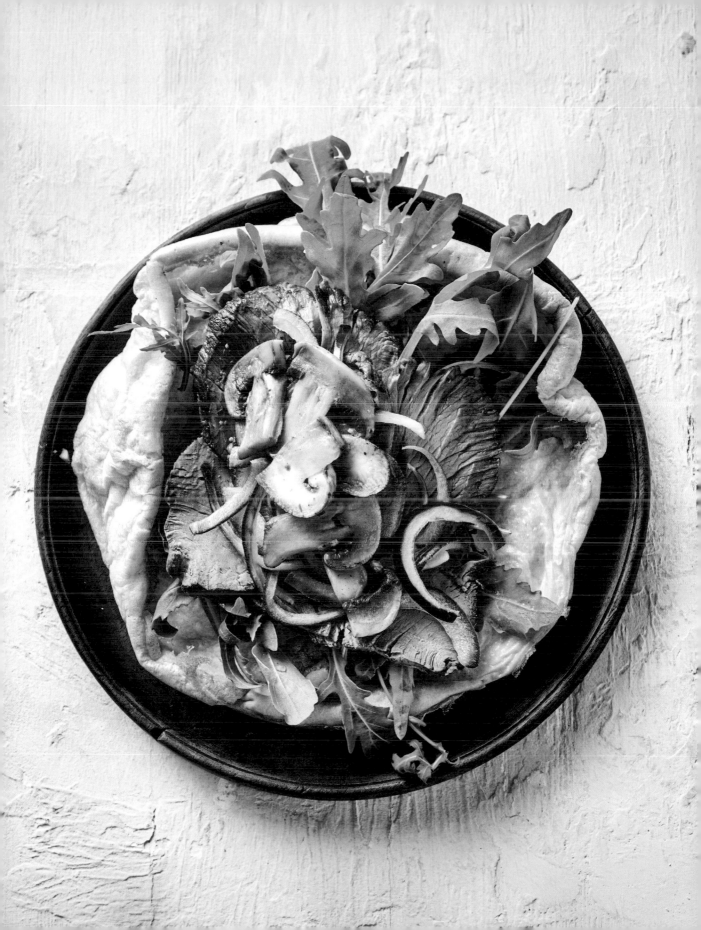

LEMON *and* THYME
ROAST CHICKEN

🕐 **5 MINS** | 🍲 **APPROX. 1 HOUR 30 MINS** | 💧 **167 CALS** PER SERVING

There is often nothing better than a good home-cooked roast. The classic flavour combination of lemon and thyme is perfect for a delicious, moist chicken with homemade gravy and roasted vegetables. It will tempt you into a mid-week roast more often than usual! Removing the skin after cooking will still leave you with the delicious flavours that will have soaked into the meat, while reducing your intake of fats.

Everyday Light

SERVES 4–6

1 large chicken
grated zest of 1 lemon (then cut the
    lemon in half and reserve)
1 tsp salt (preferably flakes)
grind of black pepper
½ tsp dried thyme (or a bunch of
    fresh thyme, if preferred)
½ tsp dried Italian herbs
2 garlic cloves, crushed
low-calorie cooking spray
1 cup water
steamed greens, to serve

Around 30 minutes before you wish to cook, take the chicken out of the fridge.

Preheat the oven to 375°F (fan 350°F).

Place the chicken in a large, deep roasting tray with a rack on the bottom. If you don't have a rack then a trivet made out of foil will do. (You don't want the chicken to sit in its own juices and fat when it's cooking.)

Put the lemon zest, salt, pepper, thyme, Italian herbs and garlic in a bowl and mix well.

Spray the chicken with the low-calorie cooking spray, then rub the herb mixture all over the chicken. Put the lemon halves inside the chicken cavity.

Pour the water into the bottom of the roasting tray and cook the chicken according to the packaging instructions until the juices run clear when you insert a knife into the thickest part of the chicken leg. (This should take roughly 20 minutes per pound, plus 20 minutes.)

Remove from the oven and leave to rest for 15 minutes before serving.

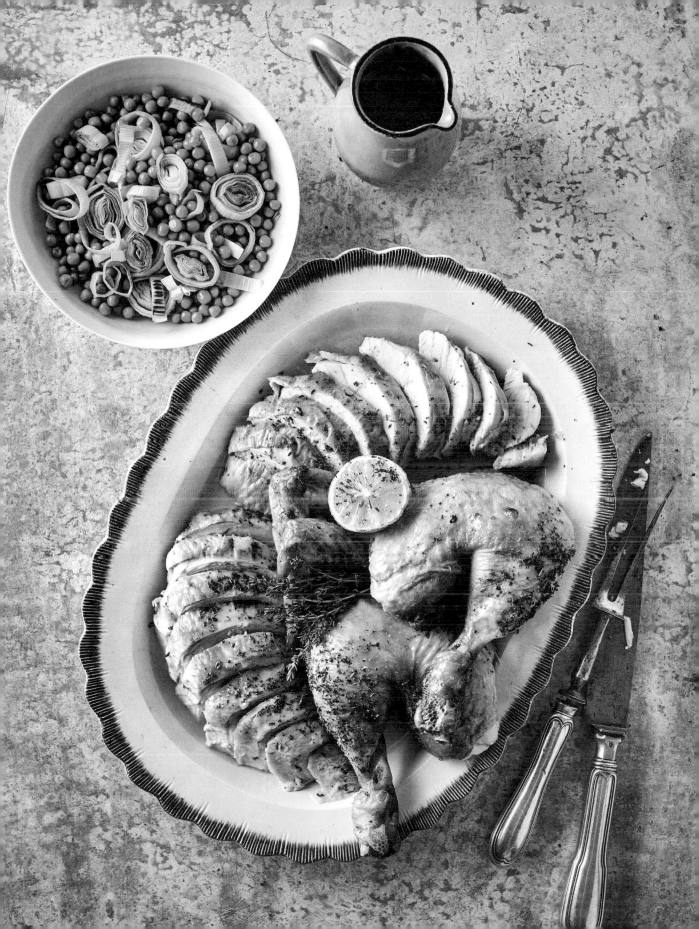

THE *Sloppy Joes* ARE ANOTHER DEFINITE HIT!

KERRY

"

Made RUMBLEDETHUMPS tonight. It was *attacked* by six ravenous teenagers!

DEBBIE

Just *made* the SPINACH and RICOTTA CANNELLONI and it was *delicious*!

CAITLIN

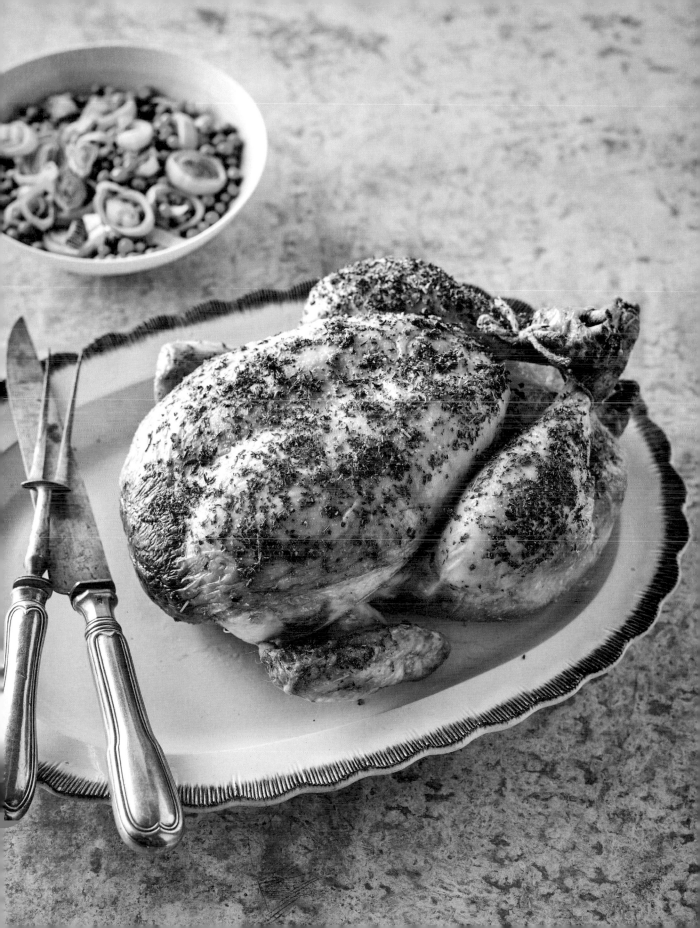

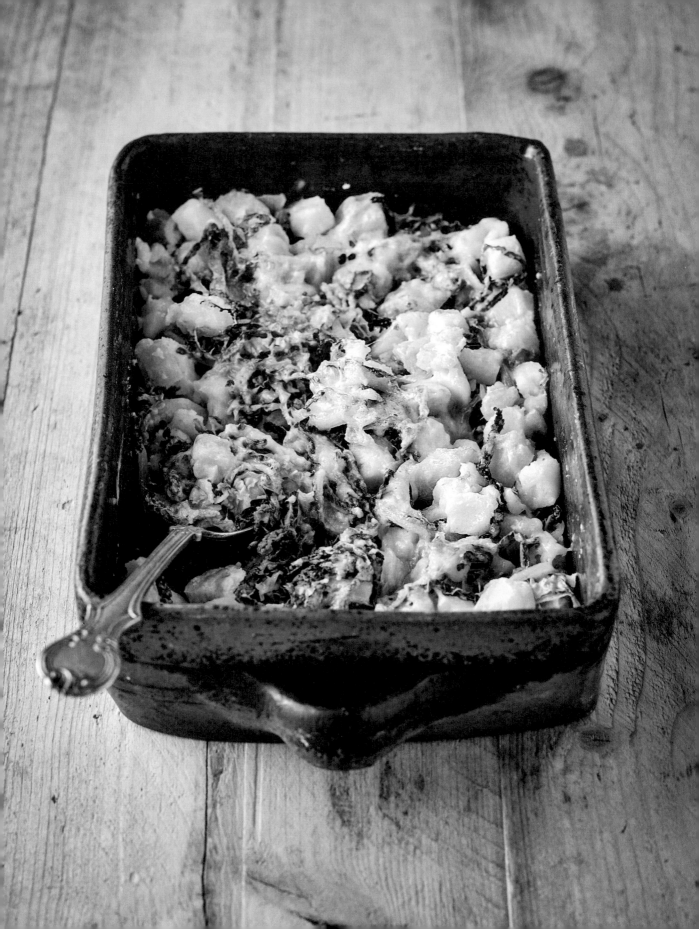

RUMBLEDETHUMPS

⏱ **10 MINS** | 🍲 **40 MINS** | 🔥 **162 CALS** PER SERVING

When we asked our fantastic taste testers to review this recipe, the most asked question was, "But … what is rumbledethumps?" Mostly heard of "Up North," it's a Scottish version of the Irish colcannon, or the English bubble and squeak. Why is it called Rumbledethumps in this book? Because we're northerners, of course!

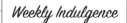

Weekly Indulgence

SERVES 4

14 oz medium potatoes, peeled
   and diced
7 oz rutabaga, peeled and diced
low-calorie cooking spray
½ small onion, thinly sliced
1⅓ cup green or white cabbage,
   thinly sliced
sea salt and freshly ground
   black pepper
1 medium egg yolk
⅓ cup grated reduced-fat Cheddar

Cook the diced potato and rutabaga in a pan of boiling salted water until soft, then drain and set aside.

Preheat the oven to 400°F (fan 375°F).

Spray a large frying pan with some low-calorie cooking spray and place over a medium heat. Add the onion and cabbage and cook for 3–4 minutes until they start to soften slightly, then add them to the cooked potato and rutabaga and mash roughly with a fork or spoon. You want to leave it a bit chunky.

Season well with salt and pepper and stir in the egg yolk. Place in an ovenproof dish, sprinkle the grated cheese evenly over the top, and cook in the oven for 15–20 minutes, or until the cheese is melted and golden brown.

Remove from the oven and serve.

CHICKEN, HAM
and LEEK PIE

🕐 **5 MINS** | 🍲 **30 MINS** | 🔥 **301 CALS** PER SERVING

With a few simple swaps, a pie is a wonderful way to create a treat meal on a Friday night without going crazy on the calories. Using filo pastry as a topper instead of dense, calorie-laden shortcrust pastry, you can re-create the flavour and texture of a classic pie. The low-fat cream cheese blends with the other ingredients to create a gorgeous, creamy sauce, perfect for this dish. Serve with a green salad or some seasonal steamed vegetables.

Weekly Indulgence

SERVES 4

low-calorie cooking spray
1 large leek, trimmed, washed and sliced
½ onion, finely chopped
1 lb 2 oz chicken breast (skin and visible fat removed), diced
2 tsp English mustard powder
1½ cups chicken stock (1 chicken stock pot such as Knorr concentrated chicken stock, dissolved in 1½ cups boiling water)
1 tbsp cornstarch
1 tbsp water
5 tbsp low-fat cream cheese
5¼ oz cooked ham, fat removed and cut into bite-sized pieces
leaves from 1 sprig of thyme, chopped
roughly 2½ small sheets filo pastry

Preheat the oven to 400°F (fan 375°F).

Spray a saucepan with low-calorie cooking spray and place over a low heat. Add the sliced leek and onion and sauté for 6–8 minutes until soft, then add the chicken to the pan and cook for 5 minutes. Add the mustard powder and chicken stock, bring to a simmer and cook for 10 minutes.

Mix the cornstarch with the water, add it to the pan and stir quickly to thicken the sauce, then stir in the cream cheese, the ham and thyme and transfer the mixture to a medium pie dish.

Cut the filo pastry into twelve pieces. Spray each piece with low-calorie cooking spray then scrunch it lightly. Arrange the scrunched pieces on top of the chicken mixture so the whole dish is covered.

Place the dish on a baking tray, to catch any filling that may bubble over, and bake in the oven for 10 minutes or until the pastry is golden brown. Serve immediately.

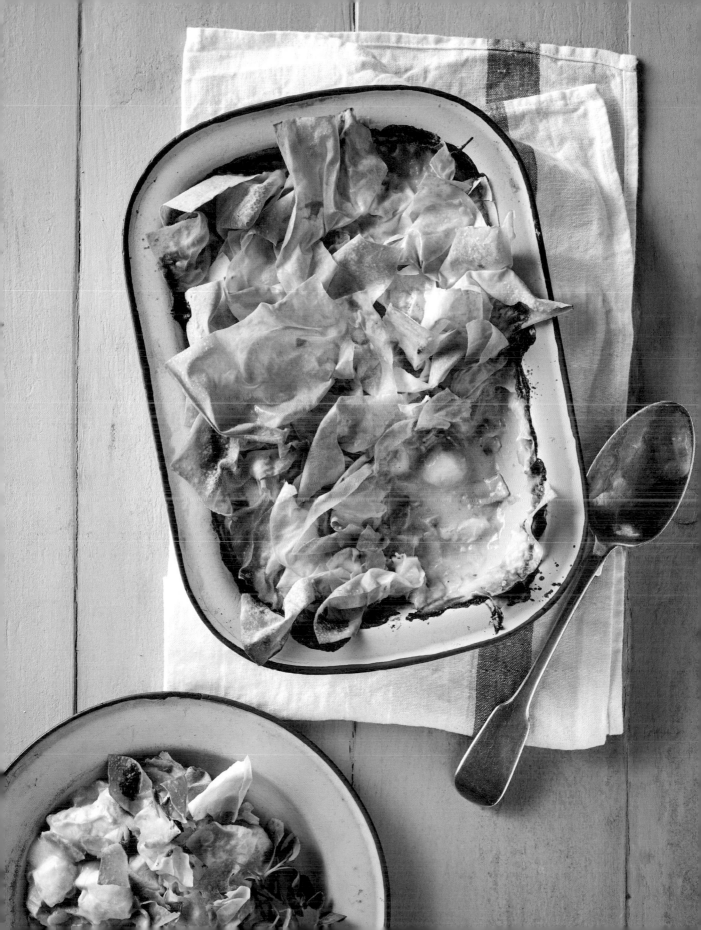

Tuna
PASTA BAKE

🕐 **10 MINS** | 🗑 **20 MINS** | 🔥 **313 CALS** PER SERVING

This pasta bake marries the most majestic of flavour combinations: tuna and cheese! Imagine a warming, cheesy tuna melt sandwich and translate that to a hearty pasta dish, then you'll begin to understand why this is such a popular recipe. Filling and tasty, packed full of spinach, this bake uses cheese sparingly but packs more flavour in with some clever seasoning.

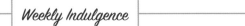

Weekly Indulgence

SERVES 6

10½ oz dried pasta (whatever shape you prefer)
low-calorie cooking spray
2 zucchini, cut into ½ in dice
5 scallions, trimmed and sliced
½ tsp smoked sweet paprika
½ tsp garlic granules
1⅔ cups vegetable or chicken stock (2 vegetable or chicken stock cubes dissolved in 1⅔ cups boiling water)
¾ cup frozen peas
⅔ cup spinach
juice of ½ lemon
10 tbsp low-fat cream cheese
2 (5 oz) tins tuna, drained
⅓ cup grated reduced-fat Cheddar

Preheat the oven to 375°F (fan 350°F).

Place a large pan of water onto the stovetop to boil for the pasta. Cook the pasta in the boiling water according to the packet instructions.

While the pasta is cooking, spray a large frying pan with low-calorie cooking spray and place over a medium heat. Add the zucchini and scallions and sauté for 5 minutes, then stir in the paprika and garlic granules, and add the stock, frozen peas, spinach and lemon juice. Cook for 2–3 minutes until the spinach has wilted, then stir in the cream cheese.

Break up the tuna into flakes in a bowl.

Drain the pasta and add it to the pan of vegetables along with the tuna flakes. Stir together so that everything is well coated. Place in a large ovenproof dish, sprinkle the grated cheese on top, place on a baking tray and cook in the oven for 15 minutes.

Remove from the oven and serve.

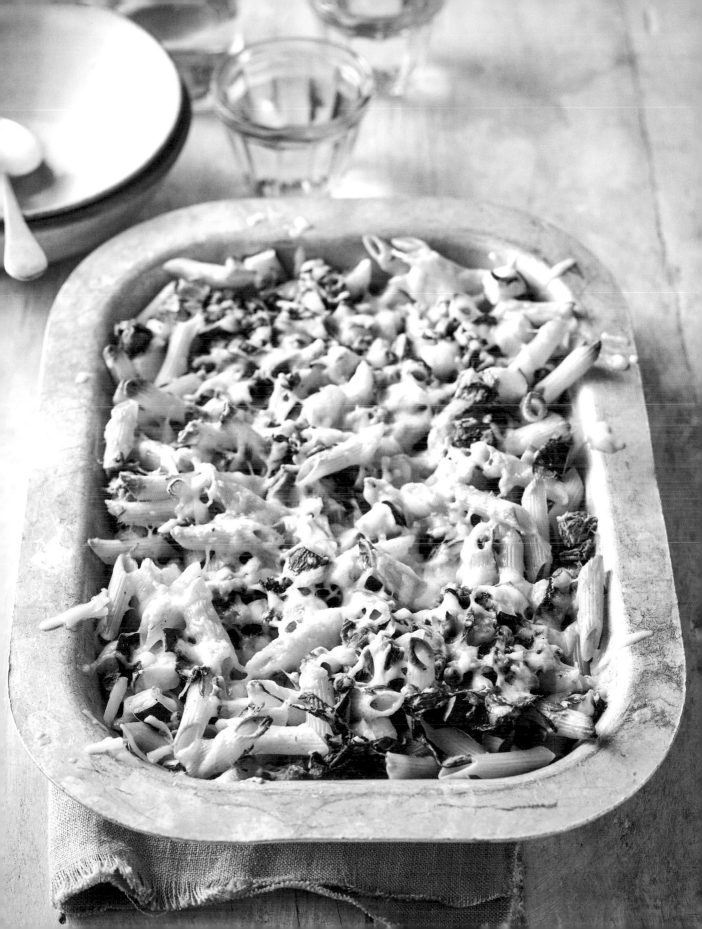

BOLOGNESE BAKE

🕐 **20 MINS** | 🍲 **VARIABLE** (SEE BELOW) | 🔥 **403 CALS** PER SERVING

There's nothing more classic than a good bolognese. Except maybe a good pasta bake. So why not combine the two in this filling, tasty bolognese pasta bake? This is a special slow cooker/pressure cooker recipe that's so easy to make in advance. It's super-simple to throw together as a no-fuss family evening meal.

———————————— *Everyday Light* ————————————

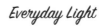

F

SERVES 4

14 oz 5%-fat ground beef
sea salt and freshly ground
    black pepper
low-calorie cooking spray
    (if cooking in the pressure cooker)
1 onion, diced
4 garlic cloves, crushed
1 (500g) carton passata (tomato
    puree; about 2 cups)
1 (14 oz) tin chopped tomatoes
1 tbsp tomato paste
1 medium carrot, diced
1 stick of celery, diced
5 mushrooms, diced
1 pepper (red, green or yellow),
    deseeded and diced
1 tbsp Worcestershire sauce
2 beef stock cubes, crumbled
½ tsp dried oregano
½ tsp dried basil
¼ tsp dried rosemary
7 oz dried pasta (use whatever
    shape you prefer, such as penne,
    rigatoni or tortellini)
1 cup boiling water

ELECTRIC PRESSURE COOKER METHOD
🍲 **45 MINS**

Season the beef with some salt and pepper and set aside.

Set the pressure cooker to Sauté/Browning and spray the pot with low-calorie cooking spray. Cook the onions and garlic for 3–4 minutes until soft. Add the beef and cook until browned.

Add all the other ingredients, apart from the pasta and boiling water, and set the pressure cooker to Manual/Stew. Set to pressure-cook for 30 minutes. Allow the pressure to release naturally (Natural Pressure Release/NPR).

Remove the lid and add the pasta and boiling water to the pot. Stir well and pressure-cook for half the time it takes to cook the pasta according to the packet instructions. For example, if the pasta requires 12 minutes on the stovetop, set the pressure cooker for 6 minutes. When cooked, release the pressure manually (Quick Release/QR). Stir, check the pasta is cooked and serve.

SLOW COOKER METHOD
🍲 **5 HOURS 30 MINS**

Season the beef with some salt and pepper and set aside.

Put everything in the slow cooker, apart from the pasta and boiling water. Set the slow cooker to Medium–High and cook for about 5 hours. After 5 hours, add the boiling water and the dried pasta and stir well. Cook for another 25–30 minutes. When the pasta is cooked, season to taste with salt and pepper.

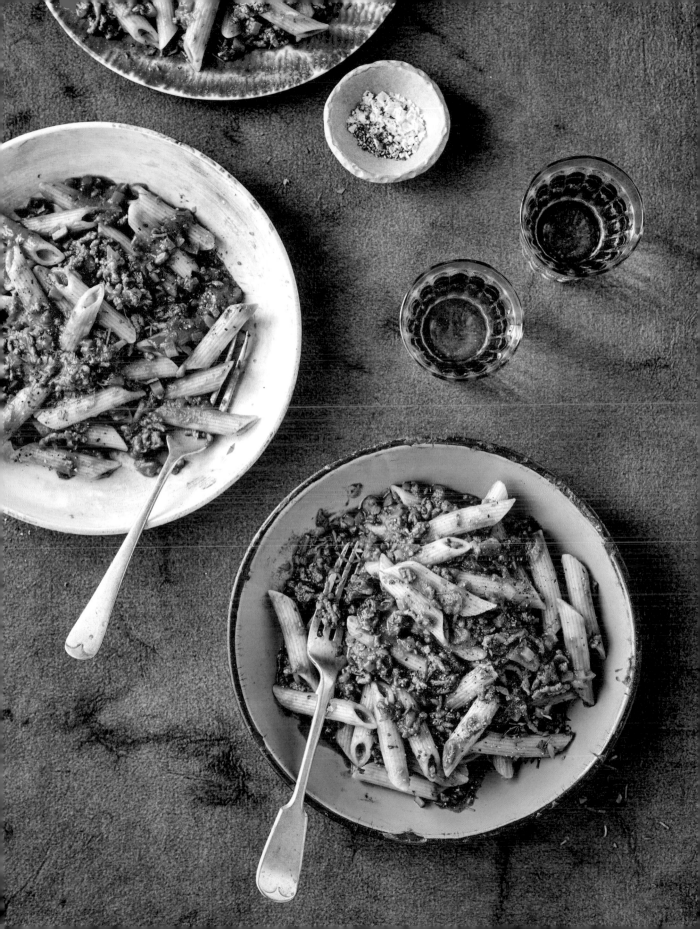

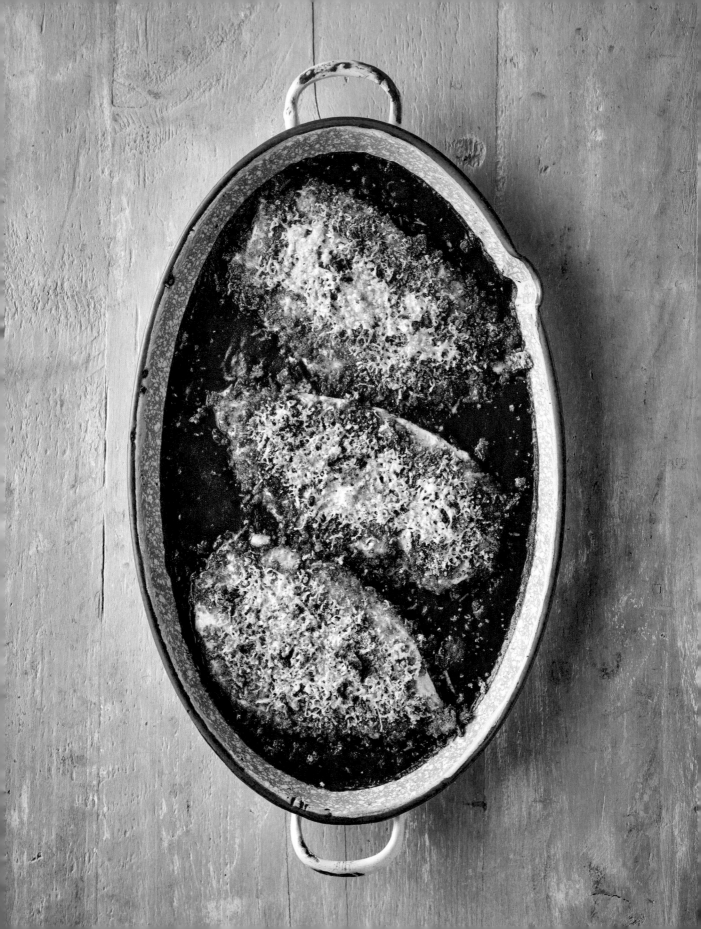

Chicken PARMIGIANA

🕐 **15 MINS** | 🍲 **35 MINS** | 💧 **277 CALS** PER SERVING

This was a childhood favourite. There was nothing better than coming home from school to crispy chicken in a warm, rich tomato sauce. This version simply uses whole-grain bread for some added fibre and a reduction in calories. Frying in low-calorie cooking spray means you won't miss the tasty, crispy chicken skin.

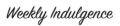

Weekly Indulgence

SERVES 4

2 chicken breasts (skin and visible fat removed)
1 (500g) carton passata (tomato puree; about 2 cups)
1 (14 oz) tin cherry tomatoes (tinned chopped tomatoes would also work fine)
1 tbsp dried oregano
2 tbsp tomato paste
¾ cup water
pinch of dried chile flakes (optional)
sea salt and freshly ground black pepper
3 garlic cloves, crushed
1 large egg
4¼ oz whole-grain bread (stale bread works best)
⅓ cup finely grated Parmesan
low-calorie cooking spray
⅓ cup grated reduced-fat Cheddar

Preheat the oven to 375°F (fan 350°F).

Cut the chicken breasts lengthways. Place each long half between two sheets of cling film, then bash the chicken with a rolling pin (or other suitable mallet) until it is about ¼ in thick. Repeat for each piece of chicken and set aside.

Put the passata, tinned cherry tomatoes, oregano, tomato paste, water and chile flakes in a large baking dish and season with salt and pepper. Add the crushed garlic, mix well and set aside. Beat the egg in a shallow dish.

Add the bread to a mini electric chopper or food processor and blitz into fine crumbs. Place the crumbs in a shallow dish and add the grated Parmesan.

Remove the cling film from the chicken. Dip a piece of chicken in the beaten egg, then into the breadcrumbs, ensuring it is evenly coated. Set aside and repeat the process with each piece of chicken, saving the remaining breadcrumbs.

Spray a large frying pan with low-calorie cooking spray and place over a medium heat. Fry each piece of chicken for 3 minutes on each side, or until golden. Spray each piece with more low-calorie cooking spray before turning. (You don't need the chicken to be fully cooked – it will finish cooking in the oven.)

Place each piece of chicken in the baking dish with the tomato sauce. Add the grated Cheddar to the remaining breadcrumbs, and distribute them evenly on the top of each piece of chicken and bake in the oven for 25 minutes until the cheese has melted. Serve immediately.

CUMBERLAND PIE

🕐 **10 MINS** | 🍲 **VARIABLE** (SEE BELOW) | 🔥 **520 CALS** PER SERVING

This Pinch of Nom favourite combines rich beef stock with sliced potatoes to make a familiar, but healthy, Cumberland pie. A few small flavour infusions, such as fresh herbs and a splash of Worcestershire sauce, alongside some easy ingredient swaps mean you'd never guess that it is relatively low in calories.

Weekly Indulgence

SERVES 6

1 lb 10 oz stewing steak (all visible fat removed), cut into bite-sized chunks
sea salt and freshly ground black pepper
low-calorie cooking spray
2 cups beef stock (1 beef stock cube dissolved in 2 cups boiling water)
2 onions, diced
3 medium carrots, roughly chopped
2 celery sticks, cut into chunks
a few sprigs of thyme
2 tbsp tomato paste
2 tbsp Worcestershire sauce
3 bay leaves
2 lb medium potatoes, peeled
2 beef stock pots such as Knorr concentrated beef stock
3 tbsp cornstarch
scant 1 cup grated reduced-fat Cheddar

OVEN OR STOVETOP METHOD
🍲 **3–3½ HOURS**

Season the meat well with salt and pepper. Preheat the oven, if using, to 325°F (fan 300°F).

Spray an ovenproof casserole dish with low-calorie cooking spray and place it over a medium heat. Brown the meat in small batches and set aside. Add a little of the beef stock to the dish and stir to deglaze and scrape any bits of meat from the bottom of the cooker. When there are no bits left on the bottom, add the onions, carrots, celery and the sprigs of thyme and cook for 4–5 minutes until softened, then stir in the tomato paste and Worcestershire sauce.

Add the rest of the stock, browned meat and bay leaves. Stir and bring to the boil, then cover and cook in the oven or over a low heat on the stovetop for 2–2½ hours. (If cooking on the stovetop, set over a low heat and keep an eye on it to make sure it doesn't boil dry.)

While the meat is cooking, cook the potatoes until they are almost cooked, but still quite firm. You can do this in the microwave (for 8–10 minutes) or in a pan of boiling water. Let them cool slightly then cut them into ½ in slices.

When 2–2½ hours is up, stir in the stock pots. Mix the cornstarch in a cup with a little water, then pour it into the pot and stir well, being careful not to break up the meat too much. Turn the oven up, or preheat, to 400°F.

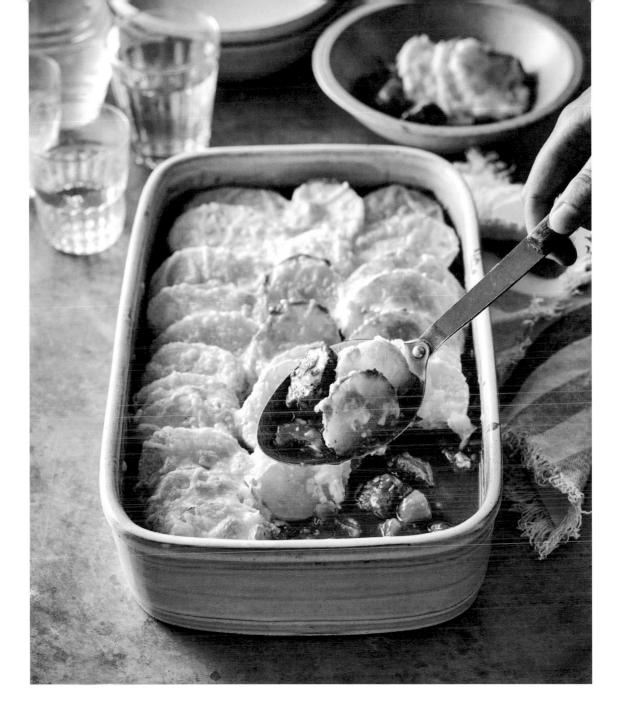

Pour the mixture into a large casserole or lasagne dish. Lay the sliced potato on top and spray with some low-calorie cooking spray.

Cook in the oven for 20 minutes, then top with the grated cheese and cook for another 10 minutes until the cheese has melted and browned.

More methods overleaf …

ELECTRIC PRESSURE COOKER METHOD

🍲 **50 MINS**

Season the meat with salt and pepper. Set the pressure cooker to Sauté/Browning and spray it with low-calorie cooking spray. Brown the meat in the pressure cooker over a medium heat and set aside.

Add a little of the beef stock to the pressure cooker and stir to deglaze and scrape any bits of meat from the bottom. Add the onions, carrots and celery and a few sprigs of thyme and cook for 4–5 minutes until the veg start to soften. Stir in the tomato paste and Worcestershire sauce, then add the rest of the stock, the stock pots, browned meat and bay leaves.

Put the lid on the pressure cooker and set to pressure-cook on Manual/Stew setting for 15 minutes.

Meanwhile, boil the potatoes (or cook them in the microwave for 8–10 minutes) until almost tender but still quite firm. Drain and allow to cool slightly, then cut into slices about ½ in thick.

Allow the pressure to release naturally (Natural Pressure Release/NPR) for 15–17 minutes, then open the lid.

Preheat the oven to 400°F. Mix the cornstarch in a cup with a little water, then pour it into the pot and stir well, being careful not to break up the meat too much.

Pour the mixture into a large casserole or lasagne dish. Lay the sliced potato on top and spray with some low-calorie cooking spray. Cook in the oven for 20 minutes, then top with the grated cheese and cook for another 10 minutes until the cheese has melted and browned.

SLOW COOKER METHOD

🍲 **6½–7 HOURS**

Season the meat well with salt and pepper. Spray a large frying pan with a little low-calorie cooking spray. Brown the meat in small batches over a high heat and set aside.

Add a little of the stock to the pan and stir to deglaze. When there are no bits left on the bottom of the pan, add to the slow cooker along with the browned meat, the chopped veg and a few sprigs of thyme.

Stir in the tomato paste and Worcestershire sauce, then add the rest of the stock, the stock pots and bay leaves.

Cook on High for 5–6 hours. You may have to remove the lid to allow the liquid to reduce slightly. When the meat is cooked mix the cornstarch with a little water, then pour it into the pot, stirring well, but be careful not to break up the meat too much. Pour the meat into a decent-sized ovenproof casserole or lasagne dish.

Preheat the oven to 400°F. Boil the potatoes (or cook them in the microwave for 8–10 minutes) until they are almost tender but still quite firm.

Drain and allow the potatoes to cool slightly, then cut them into slices about ½ in thick. Top the meat in the dish with the sliced potato and spray with some low calorie cooking spray.

Cook in the oven for 20 minutes, then top with the grated cheese and cook for another 10 minutes until the cheese has melted.

MEAT *and* POTATO PASTIES

⏱ **10 MINS** | 🍲 **VARIABLE** (SEE BELOW) | 🔥 **530 CALS** PER SERVING

We have a selection of pastie recipes on the website and they're always crowd-pleasers! By using a low-calorie tortilla wrap instead of fatty pastry, you can still achieve that golden crispy exterior. Packed full of classic meat and potato filling, this is a hugely satisfying meal that's worth a few extra calories. *(Pictured overleaf)*

Special Occasion

Use GF wraps ↗

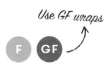

MAKES 4

1 lb 2 oz stewing steak (all visible
    fat removed), cut into
    bite-sized chunks
sea salt and freshly ground
    black pepper
low-calorie cooking spray (if
    cooking in the pressure cooker)
8 shallots, peeled and left whole
3 medium carrots, sliced
1 cup quartered mushrooms
1⅔ cups beef stock (1 beef stock cube
    dissolved in 1⅔ c boiling water)
1 tbsp Worcestershire sauce
1 beef stock pot such as Knorr
    concentrated beef stock
1 tbsp balsamic vinegar
1 tsp dried thyme
2 large potatoes, peeled and
    thinly sliced
1 medium egg
4 low-calorie tortilla wraps
1 onion, sliced

OVEN METHOD
🍲 **3 HOURS**

Season the meat with plenty of salt and pepper

Preheat the oven to 325°F (fan 300°F).

Place all the ingredients (except the egg, tortilla wraps and sliced onion) in an ovenproof casserole dish. Cover and transfer it to the oven and cook for 2–2½ hours.

During the last hour remove the lid, to allow moisture to escape and the sauce to thicken. Allow to cool.

Turn the oven up to 350°F (fan 325°F).

Beat the egg. Add a few spoonfuls of meat onto one half of a tortilla wrap but be careful not to over-fill the pasties or they won't seal, or may leak when cooking. Top with some sliced onion.

Brush some beaten egg around the edge of the wrap and fold the wrap over. Press the edge down firmly with a fork and brush the top with the beaten egg. Repeat with the remaining three wraps.

Place the pasties on a baking tray and bake for 15–20 minutes until golden. Serve with your choice of accompaniment.

More methods overleaf …

ELECTRIC PRESSURE COOKER METHOD

🍲 1 HOUR 10 MINS

Season the meat with plenty of salt and pepper.

Set the pressure cooker to Sauté and spray it with low-calorie cooking spray. Add the meat and brown it on all sides, then remove and set aside.

Deglaze the pressure cooker with some of the stock and Worcestershire sauce. Add the shallots, carrots and mushrooms to the pressure cooker, and fry for 3–4 minutes until the shallots begin to colour. Add the meat and the rest of the ingredients (except the egg, tortilla wraps and sliced onion) and pressure-cook on Manual/Stew setting for 40 minutes. Allow the pressure cooker to release the pressure naturally (Natural Pressure Release/ NPR). Remove the lid and set the pressure cooker to Sauté mode until the mixture reaches the desired thickness.

Preheat the oven to 400°F (fan 375°F).

Beat the egg. Add a few spoonfuls of meat onto one half of a tortilla wrap but be careful not to over-fill the pasties or they won't seal, or may leak when cooking. Top with some sliced onion.

Brush some beaten egg around the edge of the wrap and fold the wrap over the filling. Press the edges together firmly with a fork and brush the top with the beaten egg. Repeat with the remaining three wraps.

Place the pasties on a baking tray and bake for 15–20 minutes until golden. Serve with your choice of accompaniment.

SLOW COOKER METHOD

🍲 6½–7 HOURS

Season the meat with plenty of salt and pepper.

Place all the ingredients (except the egg, tortilla wraps and sliced onion) in the slow cooker. Cover and cook on High for 5 hours.

For the last hour, remove the lid to allow moisture to escape and the sauce to thicken. Preheat the oven to 400°F (fan 375°F).

Beat the egg. Add a few spoonfuls of meat onto one half of a tortilla wrap but be careful not to over-fill the pasties or they won't seal, or may leak when cooking. Top with some sliced onion.

Brush some beaten egg around the edge of the wrap and fold the wrap over the filling. Press the edges together firmly with a fork and brush the top with the beaten egg. Repeat with the remaining three wraps.

Place the pasties on a baking tray and bake for 15–20 minutes until golden. Serve with your choice of accompaniment.

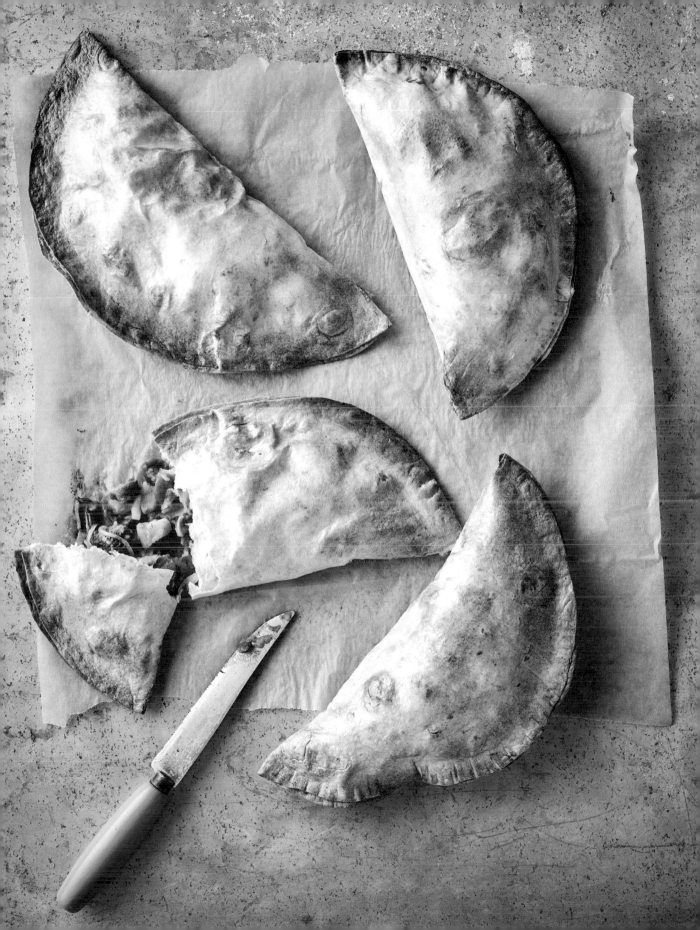

SOY *and* GINGER
SALMON FISHCAKES

⏱ **30 MINS** | 🍲 **20 MINS** | 🔥 **164 CALS** PER SERVING

These fishcakes seem wonderfully decadent, yet use the healthiest and freshest of ingredients. The beautiful, delicate taste of salmon, combined with sharp lime and warming ginger, balanced with the salty soy sauce ... you'll never buy a pre-made fishcake again.

---- *Everyday Light* ----

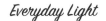

Use GF soy sauce

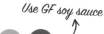

SERVES 4

low-calorie cooking spray
heaping 1 cup peeled and roughly diced medium potatoes
4 scallions, trimmed and finely chopped
2 tsp grated fresh ginger
4 medium, pre-cooked salmon fillets (around 1 lb 2 oz), skin removed, flesh broken into large flakes
grated zest of 1 lime
2 tsp dark soy sauce

TO SERVE
green salad
sweet chili sauce (optional)

Preheat the oven to 400°F (fan 375°F), line a baking tray with parchment paper and spray it with some low-calorie cooking spray.

Cook the potatoes in a pan of boiling salted water for 15–20 minutes until soft, then drain well and mash until smooth. You can use a hand-held masher or potato ricer to do this. Set aside.

Spray a small frying pan with some low-calorie cooking spray and place over a medium heat. Add the scallions and grated ginger and fry gently for 3–4 minutes until the scallions soften. Be careful not to let them colour too much.

Add the cooked scallions and ginger, flaked salmon, lime zest and soy sauce to the mashed potato and mix well. Divide the mixture into twelve equal-sized balls, then mould into fishcake shapes. Place them on the baking tray and spray the tops with some low-calorie cooking spray.

Place in the oven and cook for 10 minutes, then turn them over gently and cook for another 10 minutes, or until both sides are golden brown.

Remove from the oven and serve with salad and sweet chili sauce, if desired.

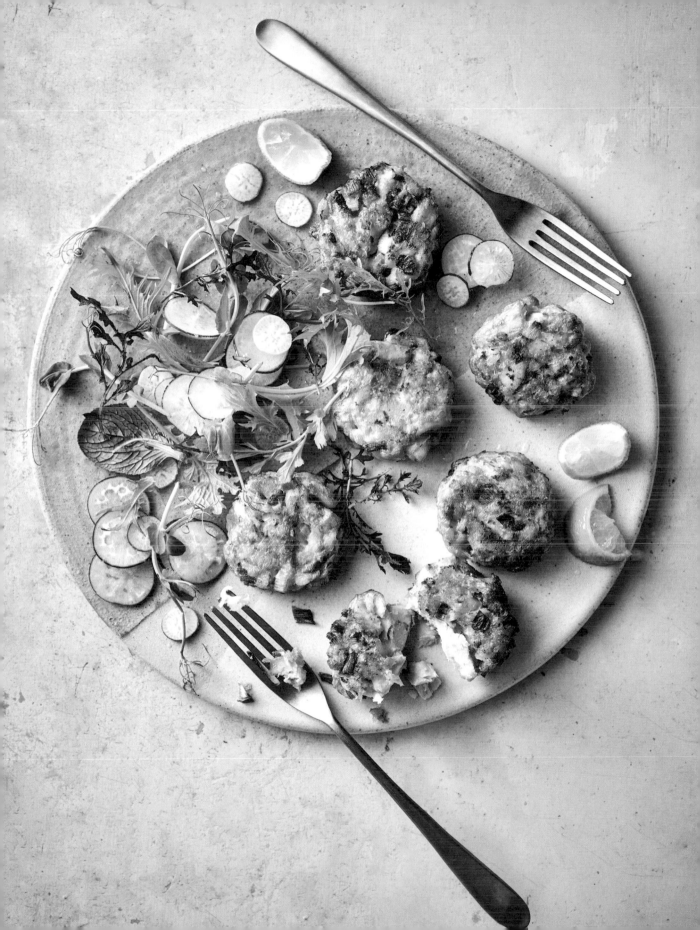

One-Pot
MEDITERRANEAN
CHICKEN ORZO

🕐 **10 MINS** | 🍲 **1 HR 10 MINS** | 🔥 **437 CALS** PER SERVING

Orzo has only become popular in the UK recently, despite being around for a long time. Although it looks like rice, it's actually pasta and it creates a great, light dish with a filling power punch. Whatever you do, don't confuse allspice with mixed spice – you'll end up with an altogether different flavour!

Weekly Indulgence

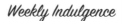

SERVES 4

1½ tsp smoked sweet paprika
1½ tsp ground allspice
½ tsp ground turmeric
1 tsp sea salt
6 chicken thighs (skin and visible fat removed)
low-calorie cooking spray
1 onion, diced
1 medium carrot, diced
1 celery stick, diced
6 garlic cloves, peeled and left whole
4 mushrooms, thickly sliced (keep them chunky)
handful of cherry tomatoes
juice of 1 lemon
2 cups chicken stock (1 chicken stock cube dissolved in 2 cups boiling water)
9 oz orzo
handful of fresh parsley, roughly chopped, plus extra to garnish

Combine the paprika, ground allspice, turmeric and salt. Coat the chicken thighs in the spice mixture and set them aside for 10 minutes.

Preheat the oven to 400°F (fan 375°F).

Spray a large ovenproof frying pan or casserole dish with some low-calorie cooking spray and place over a medium heat. Add the chicken thighs and sauté for a few minutes until they start to brown, then turn them over and brown them on the other side. Remove from the pan and set aside.

Spray the pan with more low-calorie cooking spray, then add the onion, carrot, celery, garlic and mushrooms and fry for 5 minutes until the onion is soft.

Add the tomatoes, lemon juice and ½ cup of the chicken stock, then return the chicken to the pan. Cover with a lid (or a piece of foil) and place in the oven for 30 minutes.

Carefully remove the pan from the oven, then add the orzo, parsley and the rest of the stock. Stir and return to the oven for 20 minutes with the lid off. Serve, garnished with extra parsley.

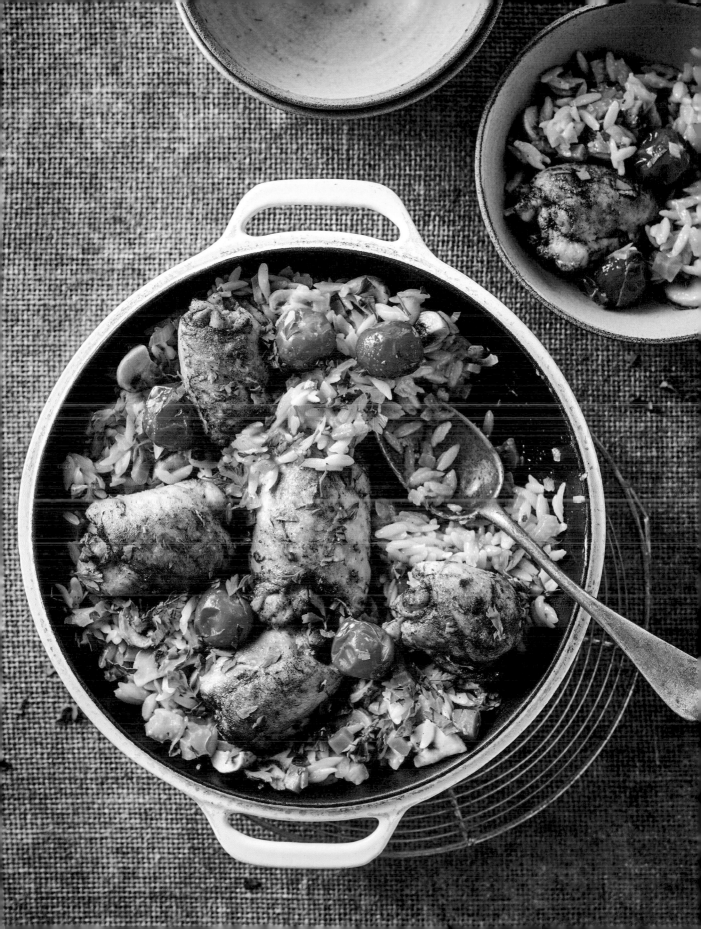

SPINACH *and* RICOTTA CANNELLONI

🕐 **15 MINS** | 🍲 **35 MINS** | 🔥 **287 CALS** PER SERVING

Usually made with a rich, full-fat cheese sauce, cannelloni can seem like an unhealthy option on a menu. However, by packing some decent flavours into the tomato sauce, and using a melting, oozing Parmesan and Cheddar mix on the top, you won't be able to tell the difference. It will feel like just as much of an indulgence.

Weekly Indulgence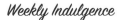

SERVES 4

FOR THE PASTA
low-calorie cooking spray
10½ oz spinach
sea salt and freshly ground
 black pepper
¾ cup ricotta
2 tbsp Parmesan (or vegetarian
 hard cheese)
8 cannelloni tubes

FOR THE SAUCE
1 (500g) carton passata (tomato
 puree; about 2 cups)
½ tsp garlic granules
½ tsp dried Italian herbs

FOR THE CHEESE TOP
2½ oz reduced-fat mozzarella
3 tbsp grated reduced-fat Cheddar
sprinkle of smoked sweet paprika

Preheat the oven to 400°F (fan 375°F).

Spray a frying pan with low-calorie cooking spray and place over a medium heat. Put the spinach in the pan, season with plenty of salt and pepper and cover with a lid. Cook for a minute or two until wilted, then drain well and set aside to cool.

In a bowl mix the ricotta, Parmesan and cooked, drained spinach. Season well with salt and pepper then set aside.

Mix the passata in a bowl with the garlic granules and herbs and season with salt and pepper. Pour half of the passata into a medium ovenproof dish.

Fill a piping bag with the ricotta and spinach mixture. There's no need for a nozzle – just cut a decent-sized hole in the end. Otherwise you could fill the cannelloni using a sturdy plastic bag with the end cut off. Fill each cannelloni tube with the mixture, making sure not to over-fill them, otherwise you'll run out of the mixture. Place the filled tubes on top of the sauce in the dish, then pour the remaining sauce over the top.

Tear the mozzarella into small pieces and scatter them, and the grated Cheddar, over the cannelloni, then sprinkle with a little paprika (just enough to add colour).

Bake for 30–35 minutes until the tubes are soft and the cheese is melted and browned. Serve warm.

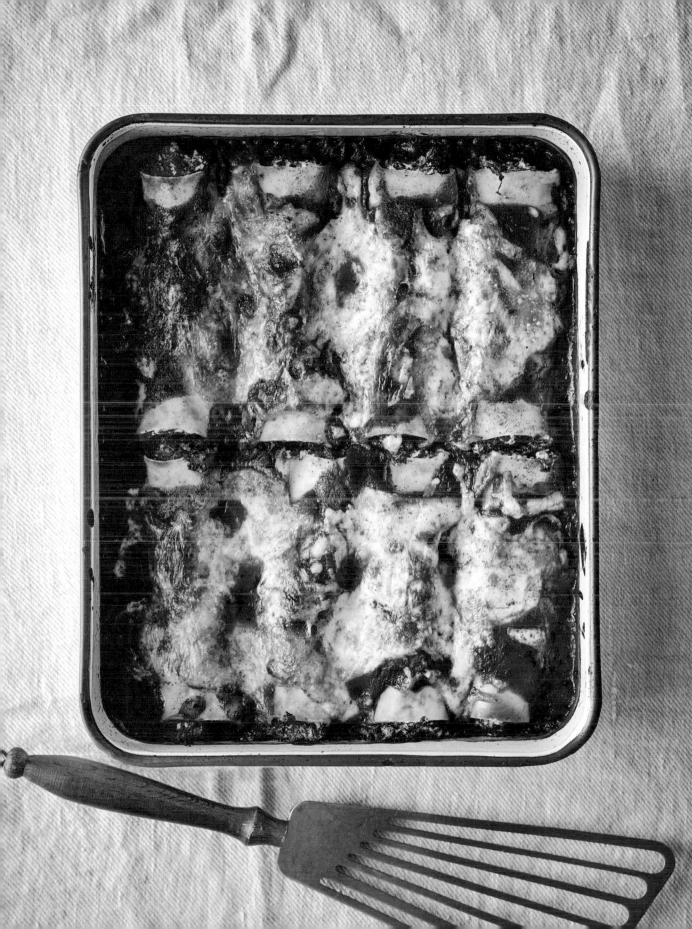

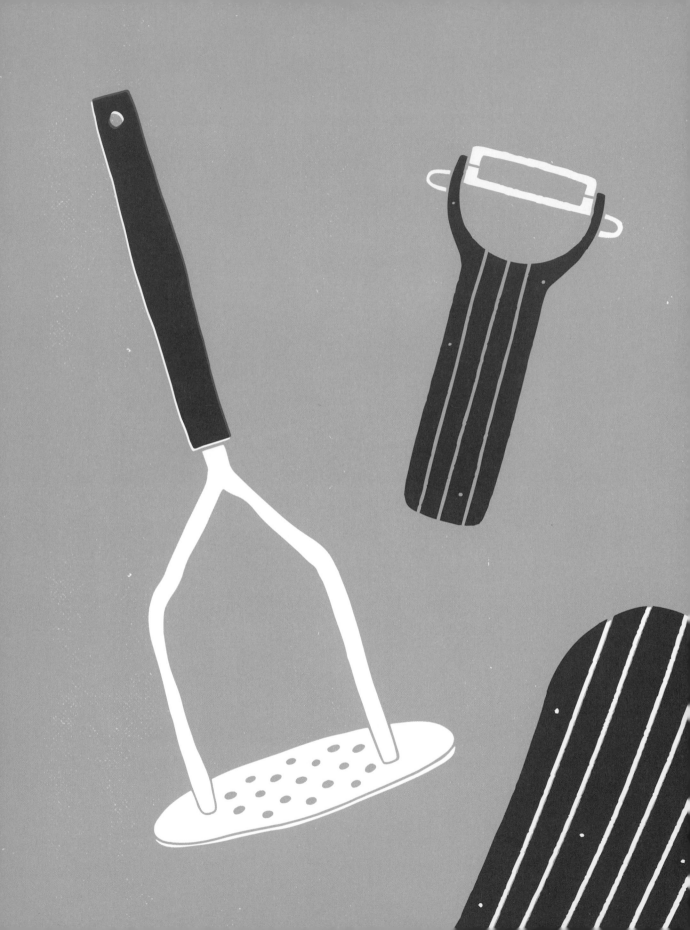

CHAPTER 6

SNACKS
AND SIDES

SWEET *and* SOUR
CRISPY ASIAN BRUSSELS SPROUTS

🕐 **30 MINS** | 🍲 **20 MINS** | 🔥 **193 CALS** PER SERVING

Sprouts are one of those underrated vegetables, sadly tainted with their reputation as over-boiled Christmas accompaniments. We wanted to create a dish that will change your tune about these little bad boys. By baking them in the oven and giving them a spicy twist we hope we can convince you to give them another chance!

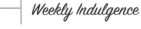 *Weekly Indulgence*

Use GF soy sauce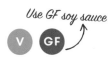

V **GF**

SERVES 4

2 lb 3 oz Brussels sprouts, stalks removed, quartered lengthways
low-calorie cooking spray
4 tsp apricot jam
3½ tbsp balsamic vinegar
1½ tbsp dark soy sauce
1 tsp garlic granules
½ vegetable stock cube
½ tsp Chinese 5-spice
½ tsp ground ginger
1 tsp mild chile powder
2 tbsp lemon juice

Preheat the oven to 475°F (fan 450°F).

Spray the sprouts with some low-calorie cooking spray, ensuring they are well coated, then spread them over a large baking tray. Cook them on the middle shelf of the oven for 20 minutes, turning occasionally.

While the sprouts are cooking, put the apricot jam, balsamic vinegar, soy sauce, garlic granules, ½ vegetable stock cube, Chinese 5-spice, ginger and chile powder in a saucepan and place over a high heat. Stir until the ingredients are combined and the stock cube has dissolved, and cook until it has reduced by half and thickened to form a syrup. Remove from the heat and add the lemon juice.

Once the sprouts are cooked, take them out of the oven and pour the dressing over them. Toss the sprouts so that they are evenly covered, then serve.

Tip
The dressing will taste very strong on its own – that's normal. When combined with the sprouts, it tastes perfect!

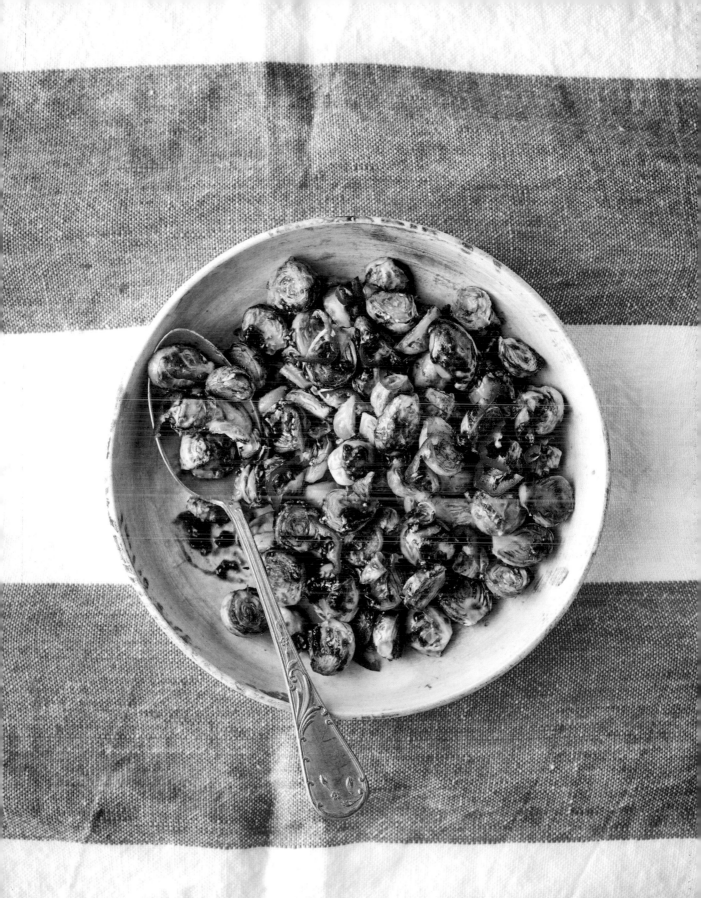

SALT *and* PEPPER CHIPS

🕐 **10 MINS** | 🍲 **20 MINS** | 🔥 **311 CALS** PER SERVING

A Chinese takeaway dish particularly popular in northern England, these spicy salt and pepper chips are a Pinch of Nom classic. They have a really authentic takeaway flavour without all of the calories. You can even keep the par-boiled and seasoned potatoes in the freezer for when you need an emergency late-night snack.

Everyday Light

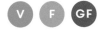

SERVES 2

3 large potatoes, peeled and cut into chunky fries
low-calorie cooking spray
1–2 scallions, trimmed and finely sliced
1–2 chiles, deseeded and sliced (depending on how hot you like it)
½ green pepper, deseeded and finely chopped
½ red pepper, deseeded and finely chopped
Chip Shop Curry Sauce (see page 208) to serve (optional)

FOR THE SPICE MIX
1 tbsp sea salt flakes
1 tbsp granulated sweetener
½ tbsp Chinese 5-spice
generous pinch of dried chile flakes (depending on how hot you like it)
1 tsp ground white pepper

Start by making the spice mix. Toast the salt flakes in a hot dry pan until they start to brown – it's very important to do this to get the true salt and pepper flavour. Mix the toasted salt and all the other spice mix ingredients together in a bowl and set aside.

Preheat the oven to 425°F (fan 400°F).

Bring a pan of salted water to the boil, add the potatoes and simmer for 10 minutes until they start to soften but are still quite firm. Drain. (You could allow the par-boiled potatoes to cool, season with the spice mix, then freeze them. They will be ready to cook from frozen at a later date.)

Spray a baking tray with low-calorie cooking spray. Spread the potatoes out on the tray and spray them with more low-calorie cooking spray. Sprinkle them with a little of the spice mix, place in the oven and cook for 15–20 minutes until they are soft and starting to colour.

Spray a frying pan generously with low-calorie cooking spray, add the scallions, chiles and peppers and cook for a few minutes until they start to soften. Add the potatoes to the pan and sprinkle with 2 teaspoons of the spice mix (or as much as you like). Keep stirring and tossing the ingredients so they do not catch and burn. You may need to add a bit more low-calorie cooking spray to the pan. Continue cooking until the chips are golden brown, then serve.

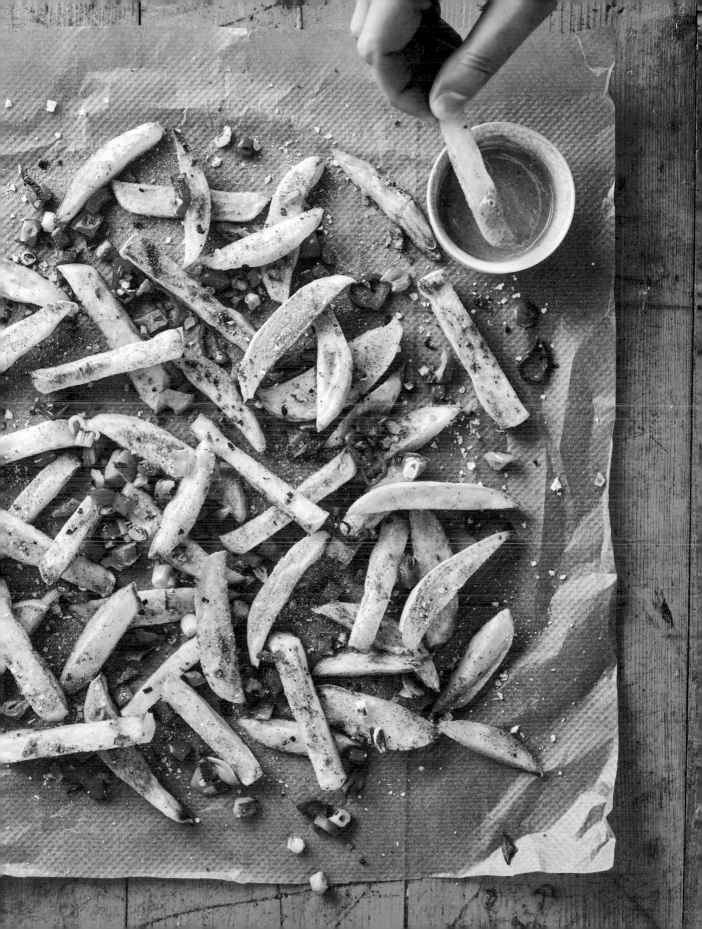

ONION BHAJIS

🕐 **5 MINS** | 🍲 **20–30 MINS** | 🔥 **59 CALS** PER SERVING

An Indian takeaway-night classic! The onion bhaji recipe is something that we have had requested time and time again. With some traditional spices and a clever trick to bake them in the familiar shape (avoiding calorific binding ingredients), this recipe has become incredibly popular and goes really well with our fakeaway curries such as Chicken Balti (page 50).

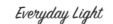

Everyday Light

MAKES 12

low-calorie cooking spray
3 red onions, cut into thin half
   moons (use a mandoline
   if you have one)
1 sweet potato, peeled, cut into
   large chunks, then grated with
   a mandoline or cheese grater
2 medium eggs, beaten
1 tsp ground cumin
1 tsp ground coriander
1 tsp garam masala
sea salt and freshly ground
   black pepper

Preheat the oven to 400°F (fan 375°F) and spray a twelve-hole muffin tray with a decent amount of low-calorie cooking spray (or line a baking tray with parchment paper and spray the paper with low-calorie cooking spray if you're making freeform bhajis).

Put the onions and sweet potato in a large bowl, then add the beaten eggs, spices and salt and pepper. Mix well until everything is thoroughly combined.

If you're using the muffin tray, divide the mixture equally among the twelve greased moulds. Press the mixture down firmly and spray the top with more low-calorie cooking spray.

If you're making freeform bhajis, get your hands dirty and roll the mixture into twelve rough balls. Space them out on the lined baking tray so that they're not touching each other, then spray again with low-calorie cooking spray.

Bake the bhajis in the oven for 20–30 minutes, depending on size.

About halfway through, turn them over using a spatula and spray again with low-calorie cooking spray. If you want them to be crisp, broil them for a few minutes once they're cooked. Serve and enjoy.

Tip
Be sure to follow the product safety instructions carefully if using a mandoline, to avoid injury.

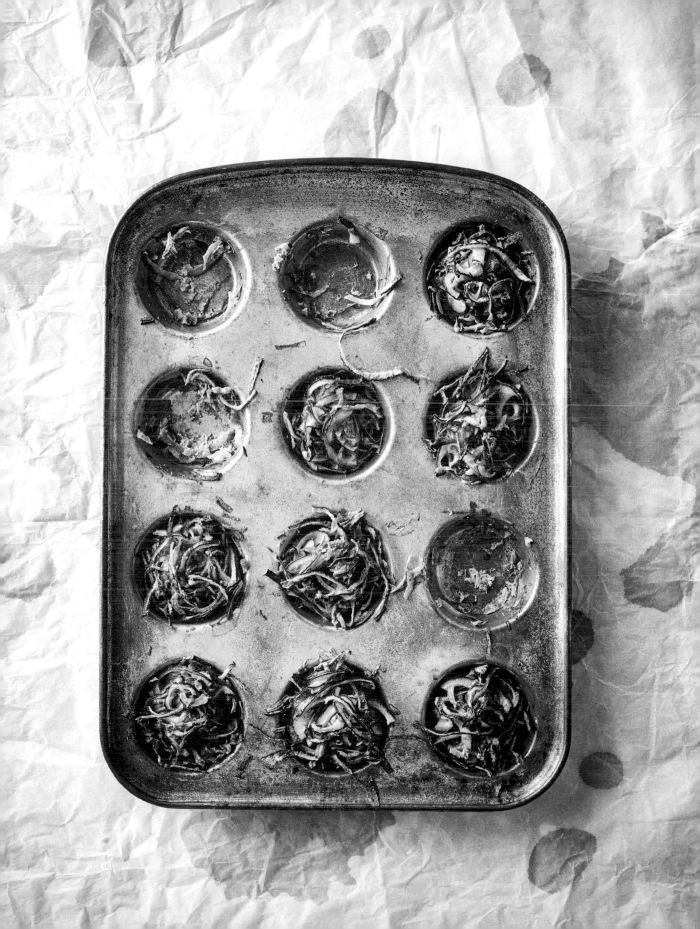

BALSAMIC *and* RED ONION GRAVY

🕐 **5 MINS** | 🍲 **25 MINS** | 🔥 **88 CALS** PER SERVING

This gravy is so versatile. Serve it with dishes such as a classic roast or a family favourite such as sausage and mash. Adding balsamic vinegar gives the gravy a real depth of flavour that will make it an instant hit.

― *Everyday Light* ―

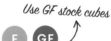
Use GF stock cubes

F **GF**

SERVES 4

1 medium carrot, roughly chopped
½ onion, diced
1 medium potato, peeled and roughly chopped
2½ cups water
low-calorie cooking spray
2½ red onions, sliced
3 tbsp balsamic vinegar
2 beef stock pots such as Knorr concentrated beef stock
4 drops of gravy browning

Put the carrot, diced onion and potato in a saucepan and add the water. Bring to the boil and simmer, uncovered, for about 25 minutes or until the vegetables are cooked. The water should reduce by quite a bit.

Meanwhile, spray a frying pan with a little low-calorie cooking spray and place over a medium heat. Add the sliced red onions and cook for 4–5 minutes until softened. Add half the balsamic vinegar and cook for a few more minutes, then remove from the heat and set aside.

Add the stock pots and gravy browning to the pan with the vegetables. Allow the stock to dissolve, then blitz using a stick blender until smooth. Add the rest of the balsamic vinegar and the cooked sliced onions, and serve.

Tip
If the gravy seems a little thick after blitzing just add some more boiling water until it reaches your preferred consistency.

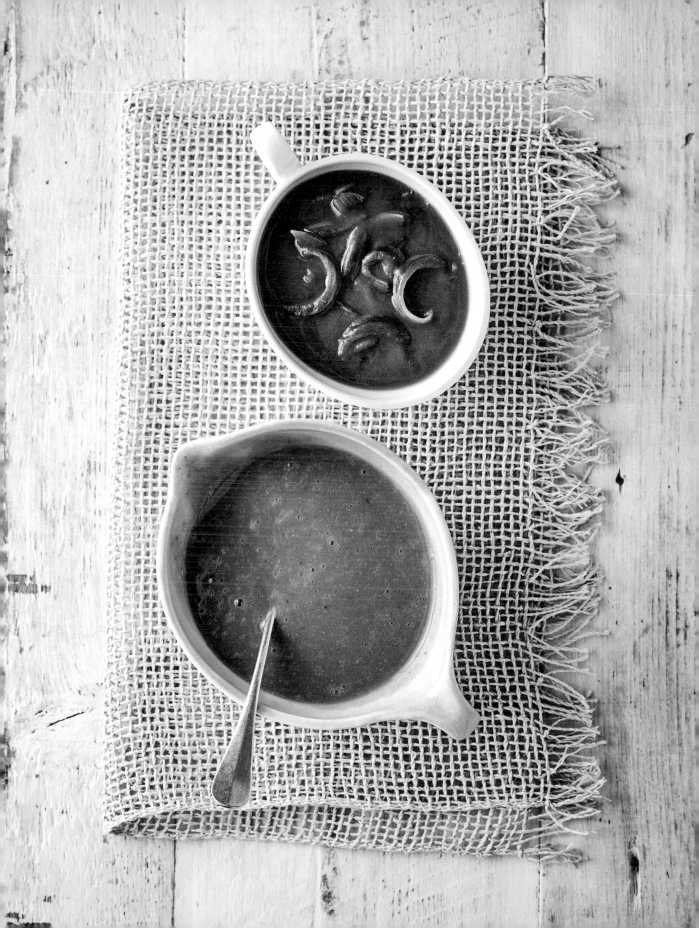

Chip Shop
CURRY SAUCE

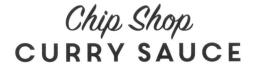

🕐 **10 MINS** | 🍲 **25 MINS** | 🔥 **96 CALS** PER SERVING

Sometimes there is nothing better than a good curry sauce, and this one is perfect for serving with chips such as our very own on page 202. This recipe uses fenugreek, which, although not essential, helps re-create that authentic, classic chip-shop curry flavour.

(Pictured with the gravy on previous page)

—————————————— | *Everyday Light* | ——————————————

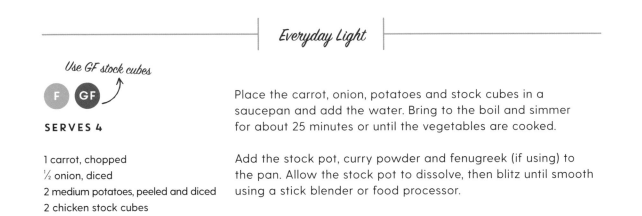

Use GF stock cubes

F **GF** ↗

SERVES 4

1 carrot, chopped

½ onion, diced

2 medium potatoes, peeled and diced

2 chicken stock cubes

2½ cups water

1 beef stock pot such as Knorr concentrated beef stock

1½ tbsp curry powder (mild, medium or hot)

pinch of ground fenugreek (optional)

Place the carrot, onion, potatoes and stock cubes in a saucepan and add the water. Bring to the boil and simmer for about 25 minutes or until the vegetables are cooked.

Add the stock pot, curry powder and fenugreek (if using) to the pan. Allow the stock pot to dissolve, then blitz until smooth using a stick blender or food processor.

EASY PILAF RICE
with CHICKPEAS

🕐 **15 MINS** | 🍲 **30 MINS** | 💧 **275 CALS** PER SERVING

This quick and easy recipe is a great way to add extra filling power. Chickpeas are a great source of protein and fibre and will really sustain you. The simple flavourings of the onion, stock and parsley make this a tasty side dish you can also enjoy cold the following day. *(Pictured with the Lamb Guvech on page 155)*

Everyday Light

Use a GF stock cube.

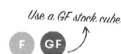

SERVES 4

low-calorie cooking spray
½ onion, finely diced
1 cup plus 2 tbsp basmati rice,
   rinsed and drained
2 cups chicken stock (1 chicken
   stock cube dissolved in 2 cups
   boiling water)
1 (14 oz) tin chickpeas, drained
   and rinsed
handful of fresh parsley, chopped

Spray a saucepan with some low-calorie cooking spray and place over a medium heat. Add the onion and cook for 4–5 minutes until it starts to soften, then add the rice and stir well so all the grains are coated in the oil and combined with the onion. Pour in the stock and add the chickpeas. Bring to the boil then turn the heat down to low, cover and cook for 15–20 minutes, or until all the liquid has been absorbed and the rice is tender.

Remove the pan from the heat, stir in the chopped parsley and leave to stand with the lid on for 5 minutes. Serve.

Kickin'
CHEESY BROCCOLI

🕐 **5 MINS** | 🍲 **10 MINS** | 🔥 **110 CALS** PER SERVING

This is such a simple and quick way to inject flavour into a snack or a side dish (we've served with Shakshuka on page 106). Stir-fried with a little Parmesan, these crisp bites feel like a proper treat. Kids and adults alike will be amazed that broccoli can become a really moreish snack.

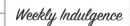

Weekly Indulgence

SERVES 2

low-calorie cooking spray
1 large head of broccoli, cut into
    bite-sized florets
1 tsp garlic granules
½ tsp dried chile flakes
sea salt and freshly ground
    black pepper
juice of ½ lemon
⅓ cup grated Parmesan (or
    vegetarian hard cheese)

Spray a large frying pan or wok (with a lid) with some low-calorie cooking spray and place over a medium heat. Add the broccoli florets, sprinkle them with the garlic granules and chile flakes, then season with salt and black pepper. Add the lemon juice and stir well.

Cover and continue to cook for about 10 minutes. Keep checking the broccoli and shaking the pan so that the broccoli doesn't catch and burn. When it is cooked the way you like it, stir in three-quarters of the grated Parmesan. Put the broccoli in a serving dish and sprinkle the remaining Parmesan over the top, to serve.

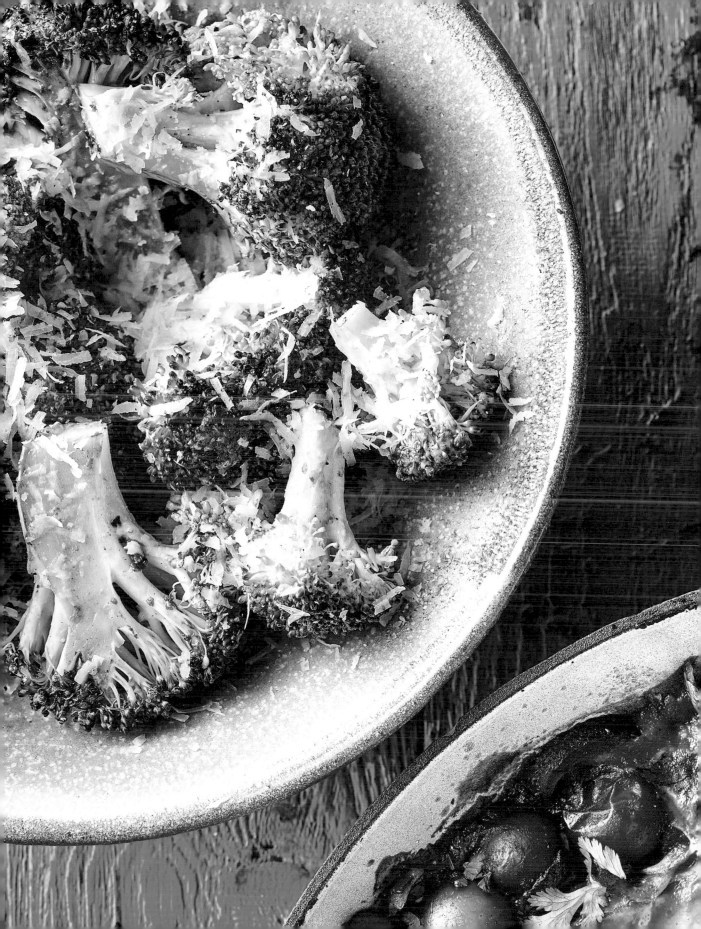

LAZY MASH

🕐 **5 MINS** | 🍲 **25 MINS** | 🔥 **130 CALS** PER SERVING

A simple technique to achieve a wonderful mashed potato taste without loads of butter is to add an egg yolk as you mash. It cooks through with the heat of the potatoes and creates a rich, creamy taste we all know and love. In this "lazy" mash, the potato skin is left on and they are coarsely broken up, making it a breeze to throw together. This creates a delicious mash, ideal for serving with slow-cooked stews and one-pot dishes.

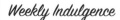

Weekly Indulgence

SERVES 4

1 lb 2 oz medium floury white
    potatoes (such as Idaho or
    russet), cut into large chunks
    (skin on)
1 tbsp low-fat butter
1 medium egg yolk
sea salt and freshly ground
    black pepper

Place the potato chunks in a saucepan with enough water to cover them by about 2 in. Add a large pinch of salt, bring to the boil and cook for 20–25 minutes until the potato chunks are soft (you want them very soft – a dinner knife should be able to cut through them with ease).

Drain the potatoes using a colander, then tip them back into the warm saucepan and add the low-fat butter and the egg yolk.

Using a knife, cut through the potatoes repeatedly, mixing in the yolk and low-fat butter with the knife as you go. You want to leave the mash chunky, with more of a structure to the potatoes – don't go as mad as you would with standard mashed potato.

Season to taste with salt and pepper.

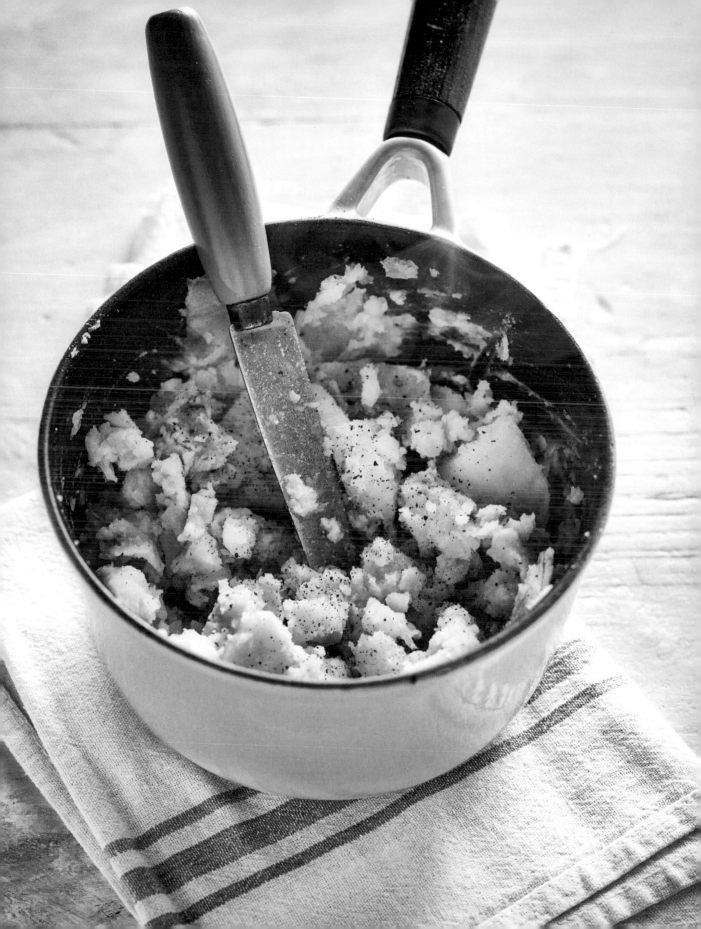

BANG BANG
Cauli

🕐 **10 MINS** | 🍲 **20 MINS** | 🔥 **70 CALS** PER SERVING

A Pinch of Nom fan told us, "I wish vegetables were tasty enough to snack on, so I didn't reach for crisps!", so we made it our mission to create tasty, snacking vegetables. And so Bang Bang Cauli was born. The smoky spice mix works so well with the wonderful taste of the cauliflower. Served with the fiery, rich dipping sauce, we really did nail the tasty vegetable challenge!

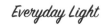

Everyday Light

SERVES 4

1 head of cauliflower, cut into
    bite-sized florets
low-calorie cooking spray
1 tsp smoked sweet paprika
1 tsp garlic granules
1 tsp onion granules
sea salt and freshly ground
    black pepper
2 scallions, trimmed and sliced
small handful of chopped
    fresh cilantro

FOR THE BANG BANG SAUCE
1 red chile, deseeded and chopped
2 garlic cloves, finely chopped
1 tsp tomato paste
3 tbsp white rice vinegar
juice of ½ lime
1 tsp granulated sweetener
4 tbsp fat-free Greek-style yogurt
a few drops of Sriracha

Preheat the oven to 400°F (fan 375°F) and line a baking tray with some parchment paper.

Put the cauliflower florets in a large bowl and spray them with a decent amount of low-calorie cooking spray.

Mix the paprika, garlic granules and onion granules together, then sprinkle them over the cauliflower florets. Stir well so that they are all coated, then spread them out on the lined baking tray. Season well with salt and pepper and cook in the oven for 15–20 minutes (the cauliflower should still have a bit of a bite to it).

While the cauliflower is cooking, make the dipping sauce.

Spray a small frying pan with some low-calorie cooking spray and place it over a medium heat.

Add the chile and garlic and fry for 2–3 minutes until softened, then add the tomato paste and cook for a minute. Turn the heat down to low, add the vinegar, lime juice and sweetener and cook for 2 minutes. Remove from the heat and leave to cool, then blitz in a blender with the yogurt, and add Sriracha to taste.

Sprinkle the roasted cauliflower with the chopped scallions and cilantro and serve with the dipping sauce.

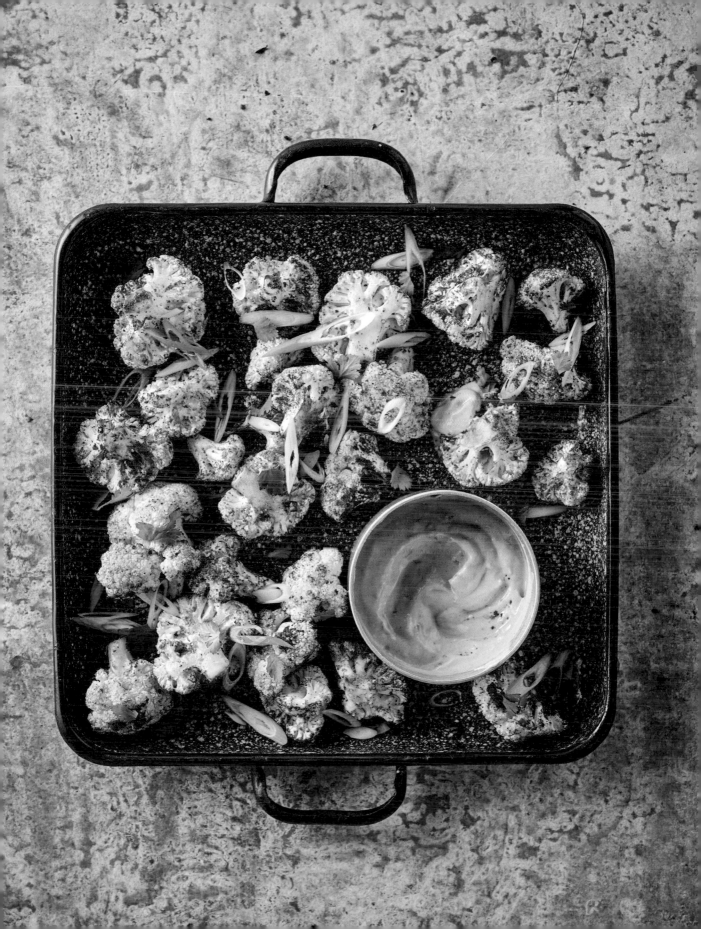

COUSCOUS *and* SWEET CORN DIPPERS

🕐 **10 MINS** | 📸 **20 MINS** | 💧 **158 CALS** PER SERVING

Why not take advantage of the filling power of good, wholesome food? Snacking on the right things can be an easy way to curb cravings. These couscous and sweet corn dippers are the perfect, filling, low-calorie snack to keep you feeling satisfied for longer. *(Pictured overleaf with the Halloumi Fries)*

Everyday Light

(V)

MAKES 20

⅓ cup water
¼ cup couscous, rinsed
low-calorie cooking spray
4 scallions, trimmed and chopped
1½ cup sweet corn kernels (tinned and drained, or frozen)
2 large eggs
sea salt and freshly ground black pepper

FOR THE DIP
low-calorie cooking spray
½ onion, diced
½ tsp dried chile flakes
¼ tsp garlic granules
1 (14 oz) tin chopped tomatoes
2 tbsp balsamic vinegar
½ tsp granulated sweetener

Start by making the dip. Spray a small saucepan with some low-calorie cooking spray and place over a medium heat. Add the onion and chile flakes and cook gently until the onion has softened, then add the garlic granules, tomatoes and balsamic vinegar. Bring to the boil and simmer for 20 minutes. Taste the dip and add the sweetener, adding more or less depending on your personal taste, then blitz until smooth with a stick blender or in a food processor.

While the dip is cooking, make the dippers, by bringing the water to the boil in a pan. Add the couscous, stir, cover with a lid and turn off the heat. Leave it for 10 minutes, until all the water has been absorbed.

Meanwhile, spray a frying pan with some low-calorie cooking spray and place over a low heat. Add the scallions and cook gently for 2–3 minutes until soft but not browned, then remove from the heat and set aside to cool.

Put the sweet corn kernels in a bowl. Add the scallions and couscous to the sweet corn, along with the eggs. Season well with salt and pepper and stir well. The mixture should have a batter-like texture.

Spray a clean non-stick frying pan with some low-calorie cooking spray and place over a medium heat. When the pan is hot, measure out tablespoons of the sweet corn mixture and place them one at a time, separately from one another, in the hot pan (you may need to cook the mixture in batches). Cook for 4–5 minutes, then turn them over and cook for another 3–4 minutes until golden. Serve up the dippers immediately with the warm tomato dip.

Halloumi
FRIES

🕐 **5 MINS** | 🍲 **15 MINS** | 💧 **132 CALS** PER SERVING

Sometimes, for a movie night or a late-night hunger crusher, you just need something quick and simple that can be thrown together in minutes. Halloumi is a great treat every now and again and holds together well for baking, without creating a melted cheese mess! Eat these in moderation with some vegetable-heavy snacks alongside, such as the Couscous and Sweet Corn Dippers (opposite) to keep it healthy and light! *(Pictured overleaf with the dippers)*

Weekly Indulgence

Use GF peri-peri seasoning ↗

SERVES 4

6½ oz reduced-fat halloumi
2 tbsp cornstarch
1 tsp perl-peri seasoning
low-calorie cooking spray
1 scallion, trimmed and sliced,
   to serve

Cut the halloumi into four ½ in wide slices then each slice into ½ in strips – you should get about twelve strips in total.

Mix the cornstarch and peri-peri seasoning in a small dish.

Pat the halloumi dry with a kitchen towel then pop each strip into the seasoned cornstarch, ensuring all the sides are thoroughly coated.

Spray a frying pan with low-calorie cooking spray and place over a low heat. Add the halloumi and cook very gently for about 15 minutes, turning them so they cook on all sides, until golden – don't cook them over a high heat as the cornstarch will burn.

Garnish with scallion and serve with your choice of accompaniment.

Tip
These would work really well with a dip made with fat-free yogurt and chopped chives!

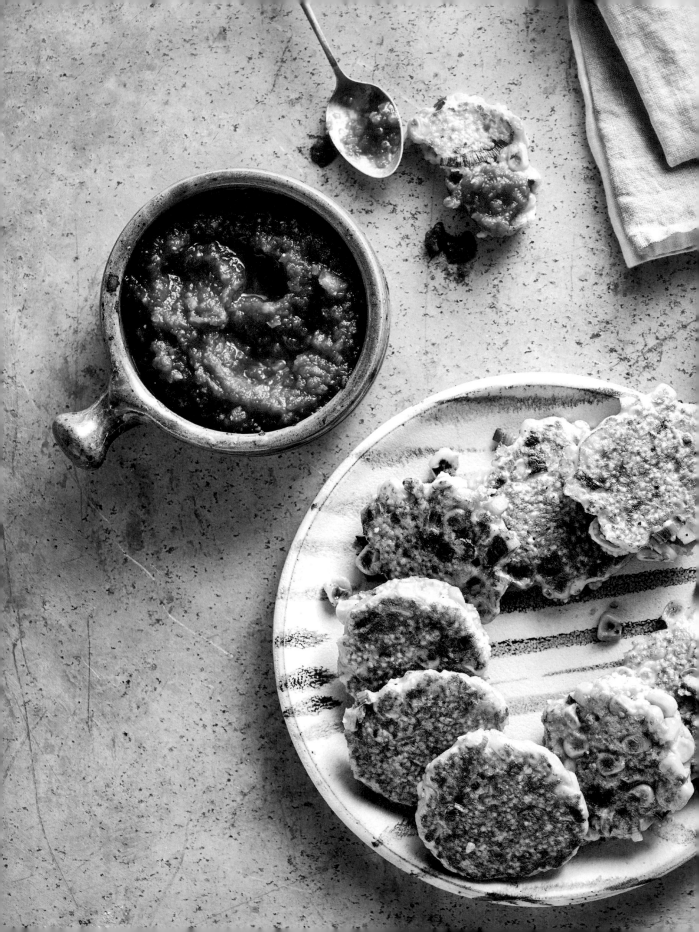

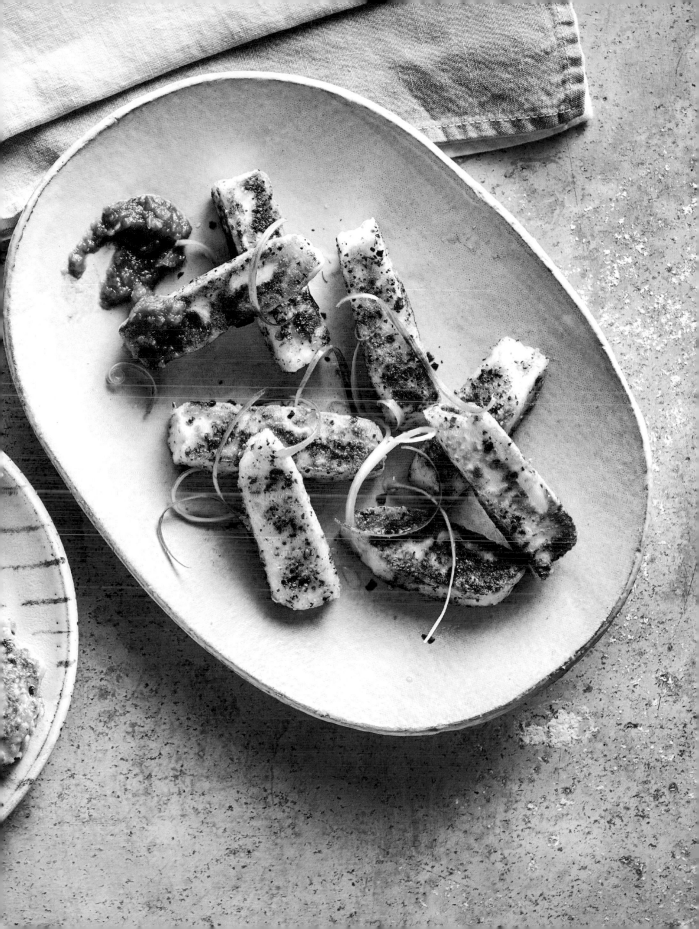

The *Roasted* ONION and GARLIC *dip is amazing!*

KATHY

> *Loved* **the CHIP SHOP CURRY SAUCE!** Really easy and great flavour. Better than the real thing.
>
> KATHY

> **The CHIPS 'N' DIPS** taste *fantastic* **and** make a nice treat on a Saturday night!
>
> LINDA

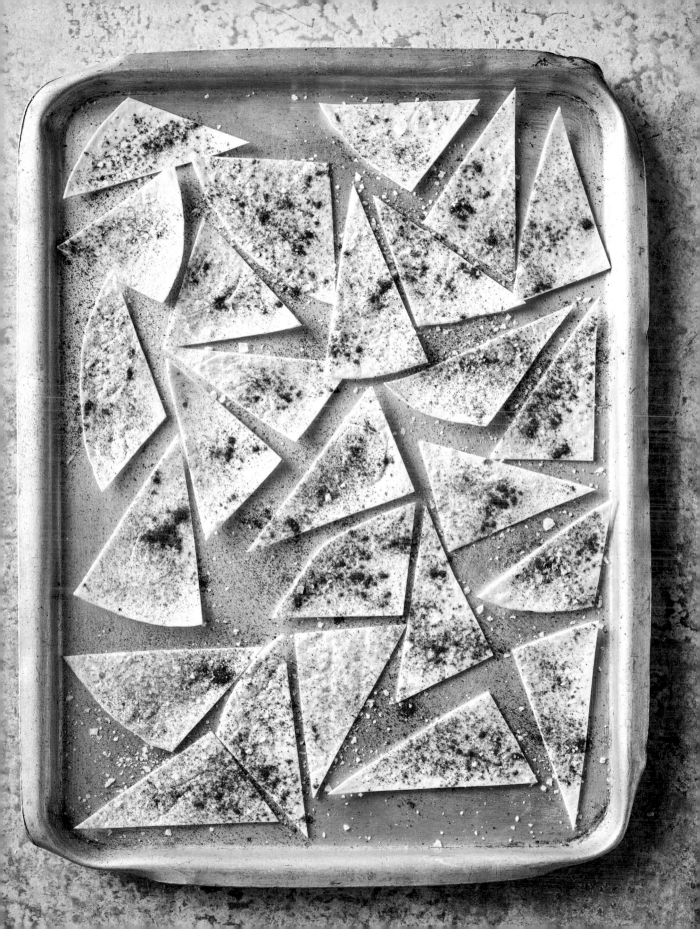

CHIPS *'n'* DIPS

🕐 **20 MINS** | 🍲 **VARIABLE** (SEE BELOW) | 🔥 **150 CALS** PER SERVING

These dip recipes are ideal for a quick and healthy snack. You can make ahead and store the dips in the fridge. Serve with toasted, seasoned and tasty tortilla-wrap "chips." A perfect, easy treat for pre-dinner nibbles or parties.

Weekly Indulgence

Use GF wraps

SERVES 4

FOR THE DIP
1 onion, cut into 8 chunks
3 garlic cloves, peeled
low-calorie cooking spray
4 tbsp fat-free natural yogurt
sea salt and freshly ground
    black pepper

FOR THE SALSA
¼ red onion, finely diced
2 tomatoes, deseeded, skin
    removed and finely diced
5 slices of jalapeños from a jar,
    finely diced
juice of ¼ lime
generous pinch of chopped
    fresh parsley
sea salt and freshly ground
    black pepper

FOR THE CHIPS
4 low-calorie tortilla wraps
low-calorie cooking spray
sweet smoked paprika, to taste
sea salt, to taste

ROASTED ONION *and* GARLIC DIP
🍲 **15 MINS**

Preheat the oven to 425°F (fan 400°F).

Put the onion and garlic on a baking tray, spray with some low-calorie cooking spray and cook in the oven for about 15 minutes, or until they are just starting to colour.

Remove from the oven and leave to cool, then put them in a blender or food processor and blitz briefly, leaving them a bit chunky.

Mix the blitzed onions and garlic in a bowl with the yogurt and season to taste with salt and pepper.

TOMATO *and* JALAPEÑO SALSA
🍲 **10 MINS**

Combine all the ingredients in a non-reactive bowl, season to taste with salt and pepper, and enjoy!

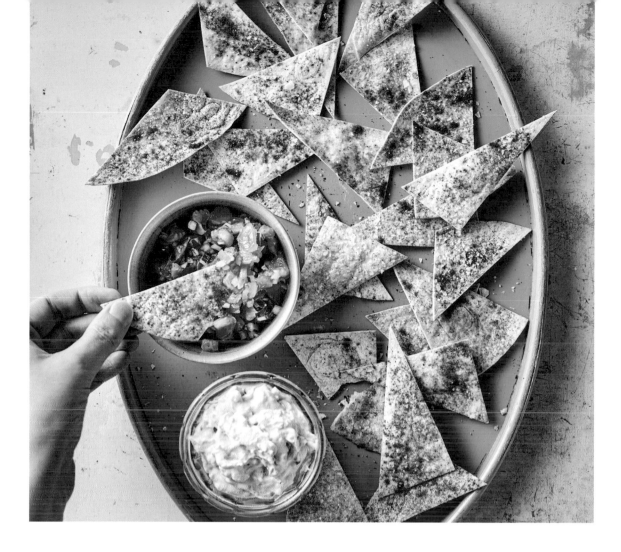

CHIPS

🍲 7 MINS

Preheat the oven to 350°F (fan 325°F).

Spray the tortilla wraps with low-calorie cooking spray. Sprinkle them with paprika and some sea salt. Rub the paprika into the wrap evenly. Turn the wrap over and repeat. Cut the wrap into wide strips, then each strip into tortilla chip shapes.

Spray a baking tray with some low-calorie cooking spray and lay the tortillas out on the tray. Cook in the oven for 5 minutes, then turn them over and cook for another 2 minutes.

Remove the toasted tortilla chips from the oven and serve them with the Roasted Onion and Garlic Dip and Tomato and Jalapeño Salsa.

SAMOSAS

🕐 **10 MINS** | 🍲 **15 MINS** | 🔥 **151 CALS** PER SERVING

Yes, you read correctly: samosas! Making a simple swap from pastry to tortilla wrap instantly brings down the calories. Filled with fresh ingredients, you'll be reaching for these time and time again for fakeaway nights (served with our Super Simple Chicken Curry on page 58), or just as a snack.

─────────────── *Weekly Indulgence* ───────────────

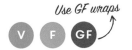

Use GF wraps

(V) (F) (GF)

MAKES 6

2 medium potatoes, peeled and cut into ½ in dice

heaping ½ cup frozen peas

low-calorie cooking spray

½ onion, diced

1 garlic clove, crushed

1 tsp grated fresh ginger

generous pinch of chile powder

½ tsp ground coriander

¼ tsp ground cumin

¼ tsp ground turmeric

½ tsp garam masala

1½ cup spinach

juice of ½ lemon

sea salt

3 low-calorie tortilla wraps, cut in half

1 egg, beaten

fresh cilantro, to serve (optional)

Cook the diced potatoes in a pan of boiling salted water for 5 minutes, then drain. Cook the peas in boiling salted water and drain.

Preheat the oven to 400°F (fan 375°F) and line a baking tray with some parchment paper.

Spray a pan with some low-calorie cooking spray and place over a medium heat. Add the onion, garlic and ginger and cook for 3–4 minutes until softened but not browned, then add the spices and cook for another minute. Stir in the cooked potato and mash it slightly with a fork or the back of a spoon before adding the uncooked spinach, lemon juice and peas. Add a pinch of salt and stir.

Brush the edges of the halved wraps with the beaten egg. Fold each half into a cone shape and seal the edge, leaving the top open to add the filling.

Divide the filling equally among the wraps, being careful not to over-fill them. If you do, you will not be able to seal them properly.

Brush the open end of the wraps with some more beaten egg, leave for 30–40 seconds, until it becomes tacky, then press the edges together firmly. You can use a fork to do this, but be careful not to rip the wrap. Arrange the samosas on the tray.

Brush each samosa with plenty of beaten egg, make sure the edges are sealed, then place in the oven for 10 minutes, or until they are golden brown.

Remove from the oven and serve warm. You can also allow to cool, wrap in parchment paper and freeze for another day.

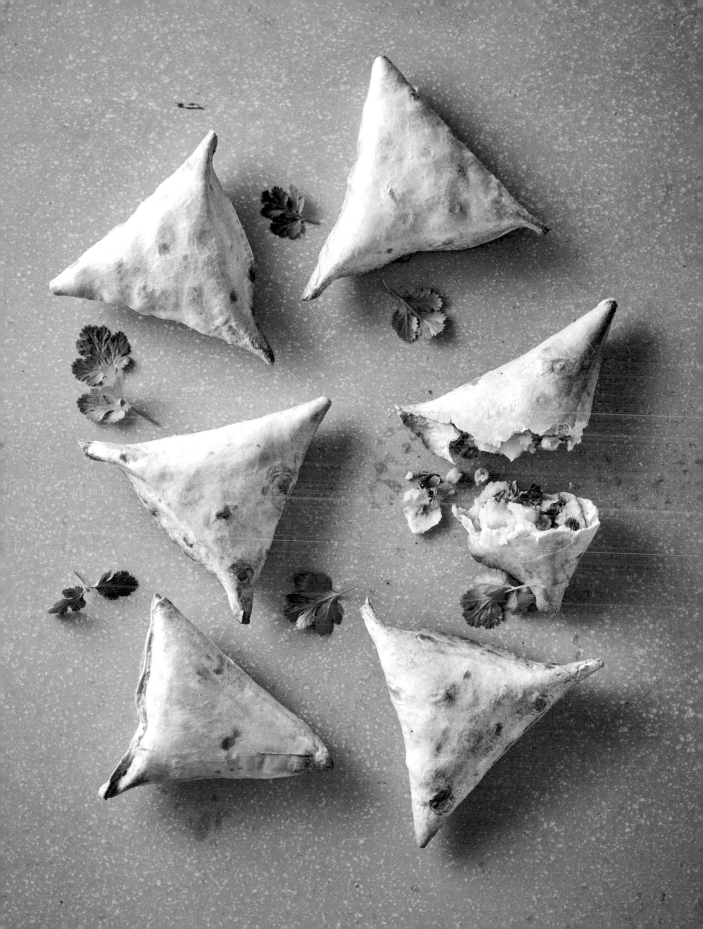

CHEESE TWISTS

🕐 **10 MINS** | 🍲 **20 MINS** | 🔥 **32 CALS** PER SERVING

A classic dinner party nibble. It's hard to believe you can indulge on these guilt free! Using light puff pastry, and mixing a little mustard powder with the Parmesan to maximize the flavour, are ideal ways to reduce the calories while not compromising on taste.

Special Occasion

MAKES 28

8½ oz puff pastry sheet
1 tsp English mustard powder
½ oz Parmesan (or vegetarian hard cheese)
sea salt and freshly ground black pepper
1 egg, beaten

Preheat the oven to 375°F (fan 350°F) and line two baking trays with parchment paper.

Lay the puff pastry out flat on a clean surface or large board.

Mix the mustard powder with ½ teaspoon of water to make a spreadable paste. Brush the paste over the whole surface of the pastry using a pastry brush.

Using a fine grater, grate the Parmesan evenly over the pastry. The next stages are a bit tricky, so there are some visual steps overleaf.

Season the pastry well with salt and pepper, fold it in half lengthways, then cut it into thirty-six strips widthways: the easiest way to do this is to cut the halved pastry into thirds, then each piece into thirds, then half and half again.

Carefully take each pastry strip and twist it several times before laying it on one of the lined baking trays. It's important not to overcrowd them, as they will puff up in the oven. (At this point, you could transfer to the freezer to be cooked at a later date.)

Brush the beaten egg over each twist and bake in the oven for about 20 minutes until golden.

Tip
Why not sprinkle a pinch of cayenne pepper on top of these to add a kick?

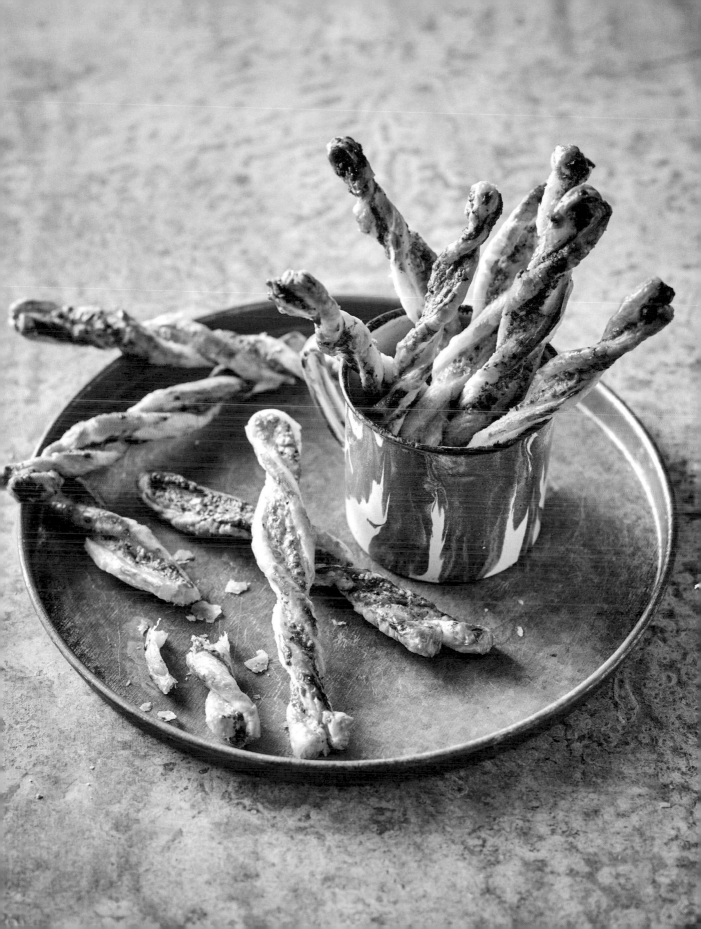

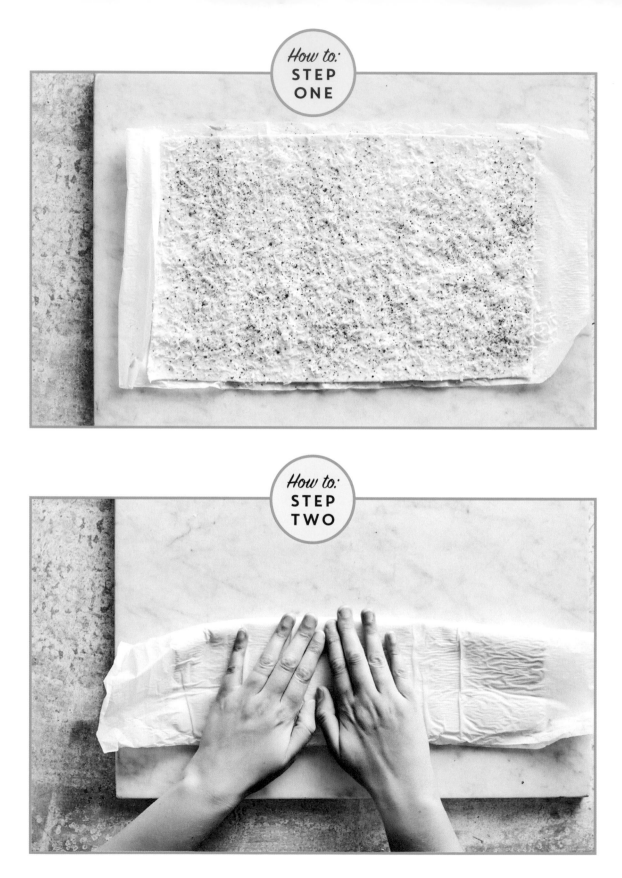

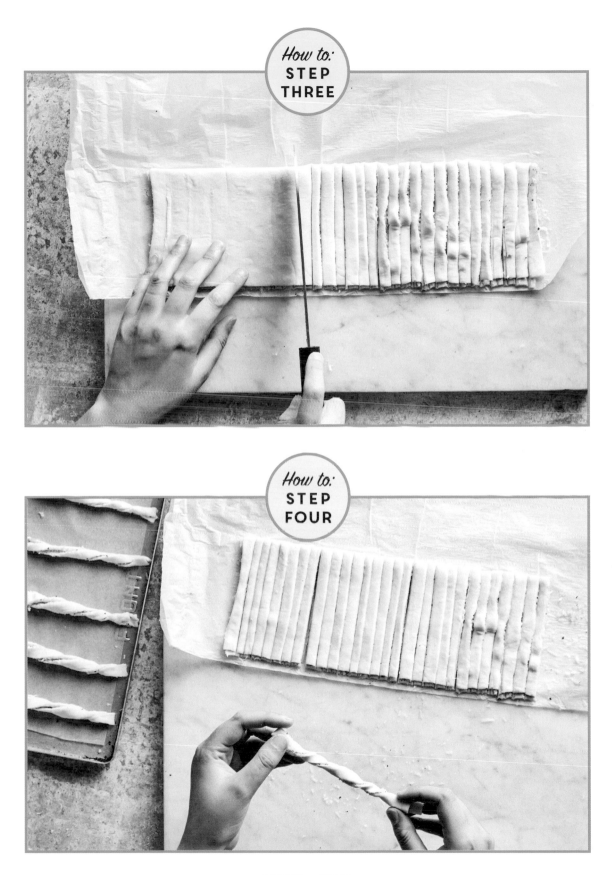

Tuna
SCOTCH EGGS

🕐 **5 MINS** | 🍲 **40 MINS** | 🔥 **208 CALS** PER SERVING

These Scotch eggs are a revelation and show just how versatile fish is as an ingredient. Replacing the fatty pork meat in this Scotch egg recipe with tuna immediately reduces the calories, without sacrificing that classic Scotch egg taste. The combination of meaty-tasting fish and boiled egg is a real winner.

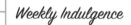

Weekly Indulgence

SERVES 2

2 medium eggs
¾ cup peeled and roughly chopped potatoes
about 1 slice whole-grain bread – stale bread works best
1 (5 oz) can tuna, drained
1 tsp chopped fresh chives
1 tsp lemon juice
sea salt and freshly ground black pepper
low-calorie cooking spray

Place the eggs in a pan of boiling water and simmer for 6 minutes. When they are cooked, drain and place in a bowl of iced water. Leave to cool.

Cook the potatoes in a pan of boiling salted water for 15–20 minutes until soft.

While the potatoes are cooking, blitz the whole-grain bread in a food processor to make ⅔ cup fine breadcrumbs. Tip them out and set aside. Preheat the oven to 400°F.

Drain the potatoes well, then mash until smooth – you can use a hand masher or potato ricer to do this. Allow to cool slightly.

Add the tuna, chives and lemon juice to the mashed potato, then season with salt and pepper to taste. Stir the mixture well, then divide it into two equal halves.

Peel the eggs carefully, then enclose each egg in half of the tuna and potato mix, making a smooth ball. Roll each wrapped egg in the breadcrumbs, then press the crumbs on so they don't fall off during cooking.

Place the eggs on a baking tray, spray them with low-calorie cooking spray, and bake in the oven for about 20 minutes, or until they are golden brown.

Remove from the oven and serve.

Tip
If you're not a fan of tuna, try a tin of salmon instead.

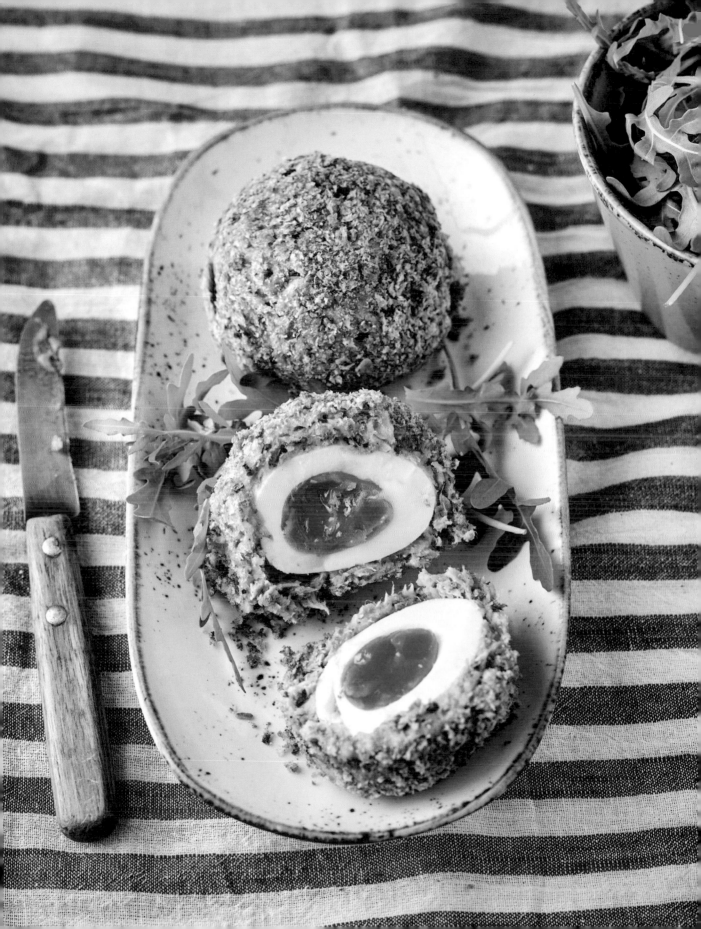

CHEESY GARLIC BREAD

🕐 **10 MINS** | 🍲 **10 MINS** | 🔥 **85 CALS** PER SLICE

This garlic bread is a perfect accompaniment for a lasagne or our Beef Ragu Fettuccine (page 151). Add a little cheese to the mix and you've really got a party going! Using some fresh garlic, a spritz of low-calorie cooking spray and switching to a gluten-free bread can make a real dent on the calorie count, but it is equally tasty.

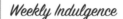

Weekly Indulgence

SERVES 4

2 white gluten-free ciabatta
1 garlic clove, peeled but left whole
low-calorie cooking spray
4 tbsp tinned chopped tomatoes
⅓ cup finely grated reduced-fat
   Cheddar
sea salt and freshly ground
   black pepper
1 tsp finely chopped fresh parsley

Preheat the oven to 400°F (fan 375°F).

Slice the ciabattas in half lengthways and place them on an oven tray. Bash the garlic clove with the back of a knife and rub it thoroughly over the cut sides of the ciabatta. If you like your garlic bread very garlicky then chop it finely and scatter it over the ciabatta.

Spray the ciabatta with low-calorie cooking spray and place in the oven for 5 minutes.

Take the ciabatta out of the oven and top with the tomatoes and cheese. Return to the oven until the cheese has melted, then season and scatter with parsley.

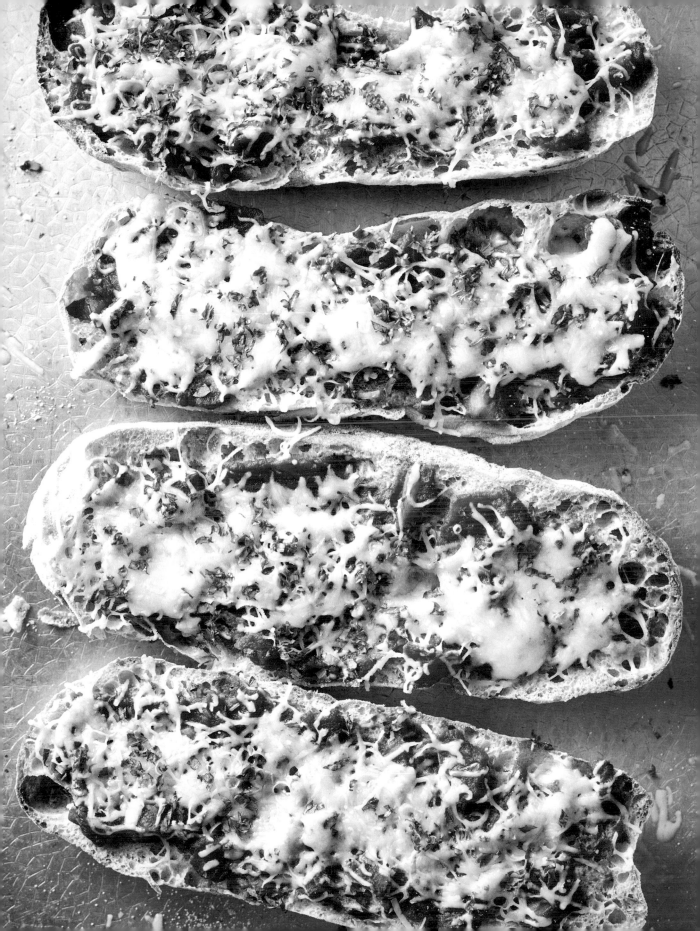

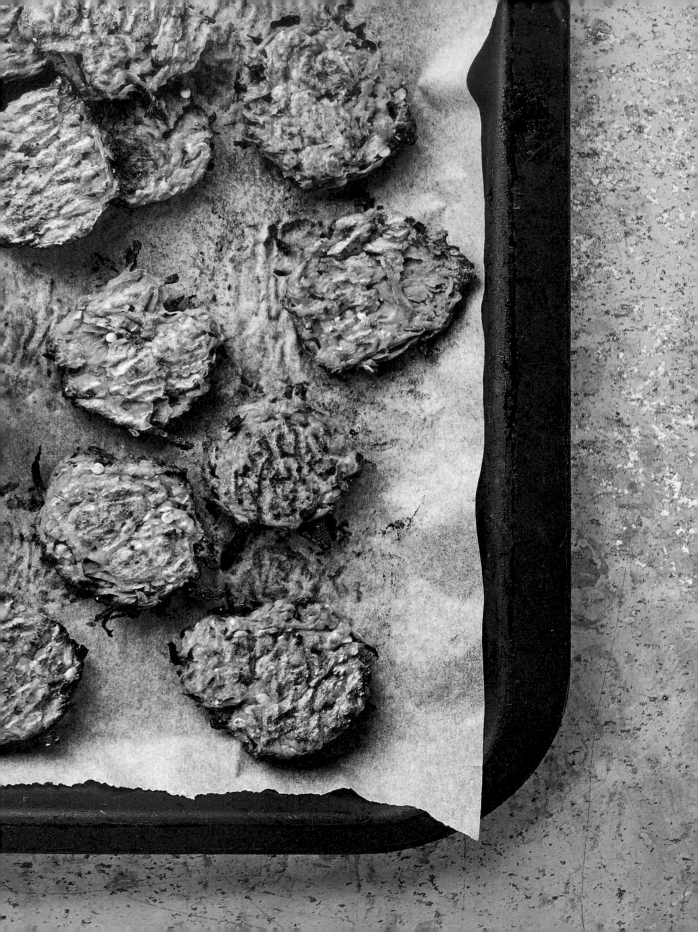

SWEET POTATO ROSTIS *with* SOUR CREAM *and* CHIVE DIP

🕐 **10 MINS** | 🍲 **35 MINS** | 💧 **33 CALS** PER SERVING

Sweet potato is a wonderful ingredient that gives these rostis instant flavour, instead of using bland white potatoes. Pepped up with some easy seasoning, these rostis are best served with a clever, low-calorie, sour cream and chive dip, using fat-free Greek-style yogurt in place of more calorie-heavy cream sauces.

―――――――――――――――― *Everyday Light* ――――――――――――――――

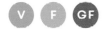

MAKES 12

FOR THE ROSTIS
1 large sweet potato, peeled
½ tsp dried chile flakes (chipotle chile flakes are really tasty!)
½ tsp ground cumin
½ tsp onion granules
1 tsp garlic granules
½ tsp sea salt
½ tsp freshly ground black pepper
1 large egg
low-calorie cooking spray

FOR THE DIP
9 oz fat-free Greek-style yogurt
3 tbsp finely chopped chives

Preheat the oven to 375°F (fan 350°F).

Grate the sweet potato into a large, microwaveable bowl, cover with cling film and microwave on High for 2 minutes. Cover with a clean tea towel and squeeze out excess water.

Add the spices, onion and garlic granules, salt and pepper to the sweet potato, along with the egg, and mix well. If you prefer the rostis spicier, add some extra chile flakes!

Spray a baking tray with low-calorie cooking spray. Take small handfuls of the sweet potato mix and continue to squeeze out the excess water while shaping them into rounds – you should have enough potato to make twelve rostis. Place them on the tray and flatten them, then spray them with some more low-calorie cooking spray and pop in the oven to bake for 20 minutes.

Turn the rostis carefully after 20 minutes, spray again with low-calorie cooking spray and return to the oven for a further 15 minutes until golden.

Meanwhile, mix the yogurt and chives in a small bowl to make the dip. Serve the rostis while they're hot.

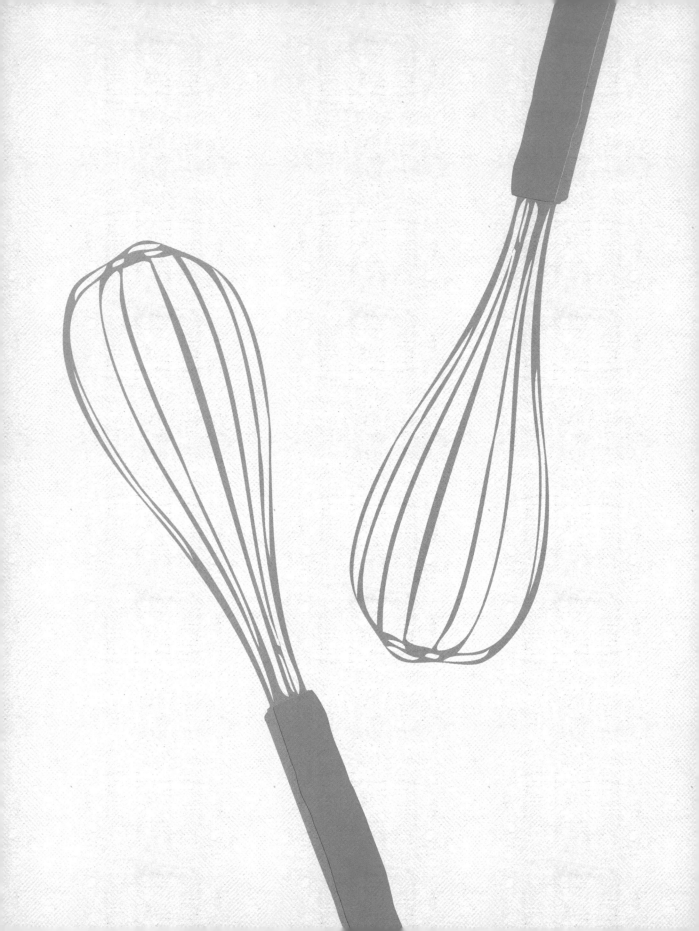

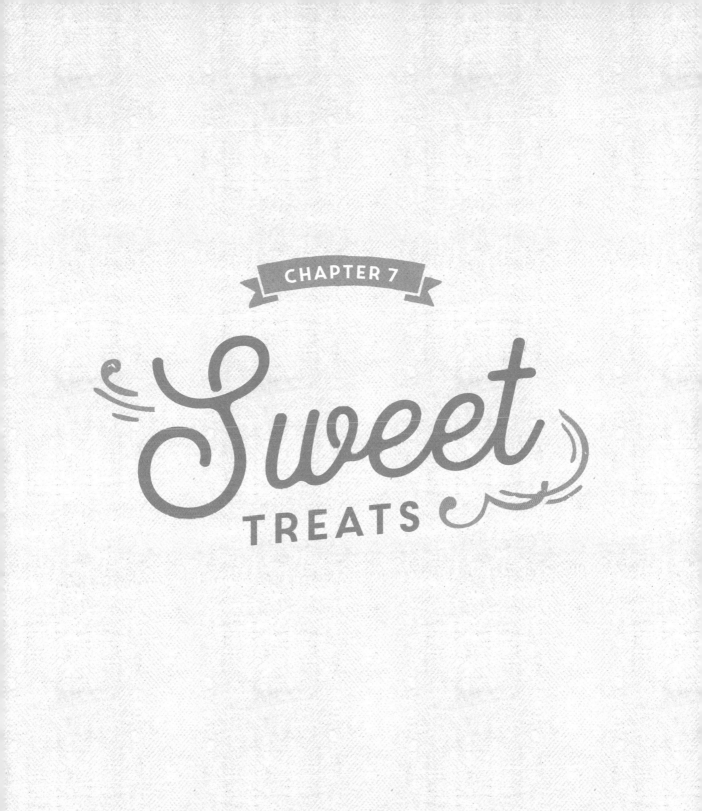

CHEESECAKE-STUFFED
Strawberries

🕐 **10 MINS** | 🗑 **NO COOK** | 🔥 **107 CALS** PER SERVING

The recipe that started it all! This recipe came about when trying to assemble some ingredients to make a healthier sweet treat to curb the craving. The blog was set up in order to share this recipe with those who may be interested and the rest, as they say, is history. It's still one of the most popular recipes on the website and, simple as it is, it's one we are hugely proud of. It's also absolutely delicious.

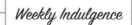 *Weekly Indulgence*

SERVES 4

24 medium–large
   strawberries, hulled
½ cup quark or low-fat Greek-style
   yogurt
1⅔ tbsp low-fat cream cheese
¼ cup granulated sweetener
   (or to taste)
½ tsp vanilla extract
1 low-calorie digestive
   biscuit, crushed

Using a small sharp knife, cut out a cone shape from the middle of each strawberry (cutting where the hull was) – you want a small hole in the middle.

Put the quark, cream cheese, sweetener and vanilla extract in a bowl and beat until smooth.

Fill a small freezer bag with the quark and cheese mixture. Make sure you get all the mixture in one corner. Seal the bag and cut the tip of the corner. The hole should be quite small so you can pipe inside the strawberries.

Squeeze filling into each strawberry and sprinkle with digestive crumbs. Keep the stuffed strawberries in the fridge until ready to serve. (But avoid keeping for longer than 1 hour ahead because they will become soggy.)

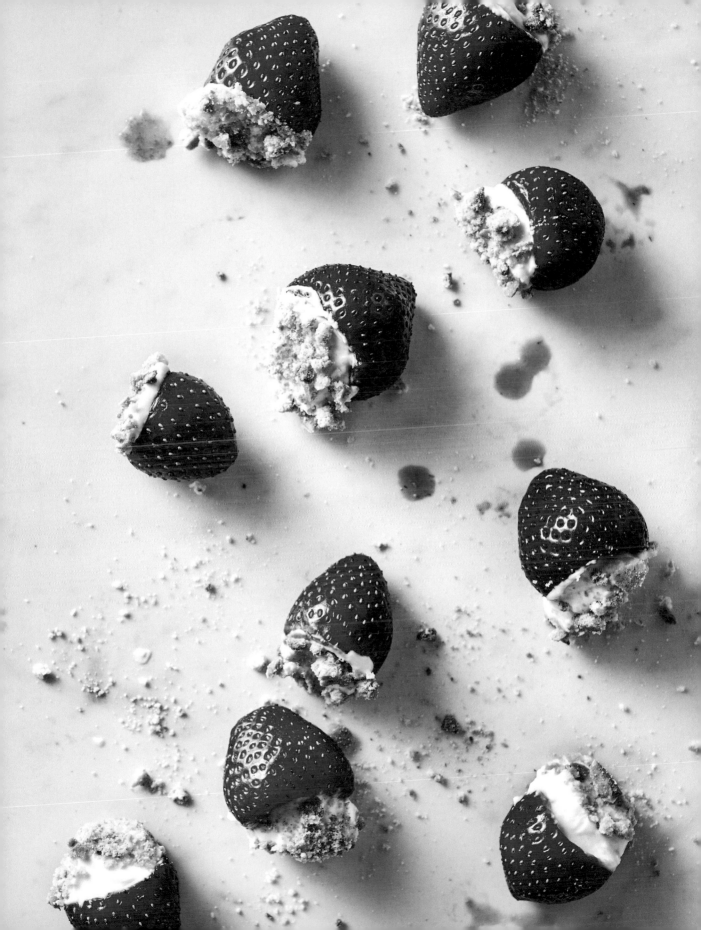

TIRAMISU

🕐 **10 MINS** (PLUS CHILLING TIME) | 🗑 **NO COOK** | 💧 **108 CALS** PER SERVING

This tiramisu is a fantastically speedy way to bring a sumptuous end to any dinner party or evening meal. Using a few simple ingredient swaps keeps it light, but it's still rich with coffee flavour. The ricotta adds a creaminess, and it's finished off with a chocolate topping.

——————————| *Special Occasion* |——————————

SERVES 4

½ cup plus 2 tbsp ricotta
2 tsp vanilla bean paste or extract
2 tsp granulated sweetener
8 ladyfingers, each broken into 3 pieces
7 tbsp strong espresso, cooled
1 tbsp cocoa powder

Put the ricotta, vanilla bean paste and granulated sweetener in a bowl and mix until smooth.

Place three ladyfinger pieces into the base of four ½ cup ramekins. Add a couple of teaspoons of espresso to each ramekin and crush the ladyfingers down to cover the base of the ramekins. Top this layer with a layer of ricotta mix, then add three more ladyfinger pieces, placing them towards the edges of the ramekin. There is no need to crush these down.

Add another little drizzle of espresso and top with the remaining ricotta mix.

Place the cocoa powder in a sieve and generously dust it over each tiramisu. Chill for around 10 minutes or until ready to serve.

Tip
This would make a great dinner party dessert! Why not add a boozy splash of any coffee liqueur?

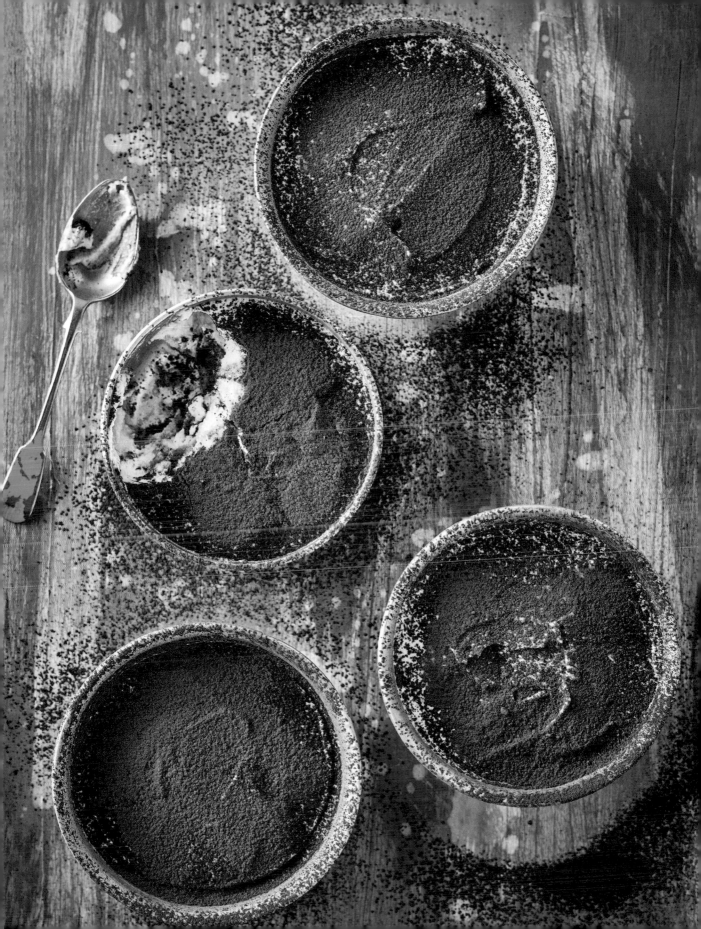

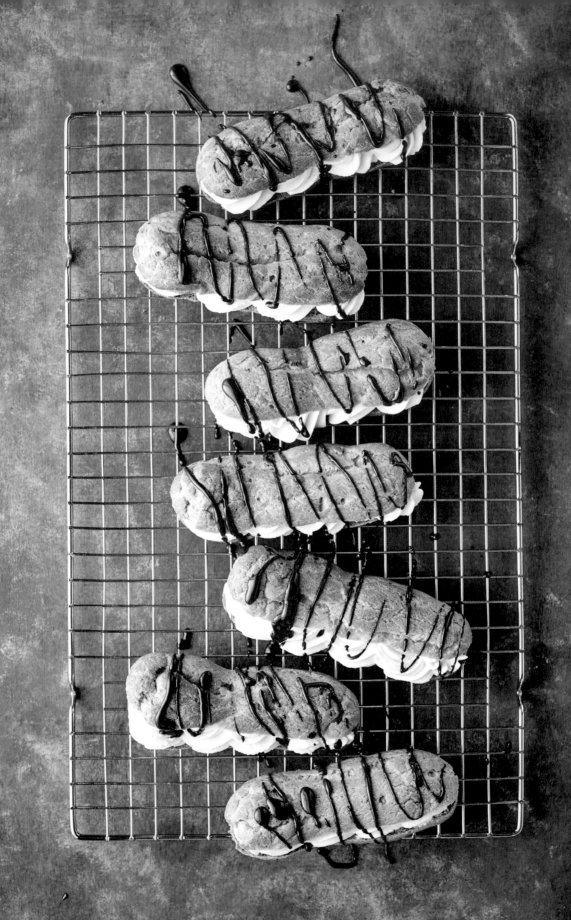

Chocolate
ECLAIRS

🕐 **10 MINS** | 🍲 **1 HOUR** | 🔥 **109 CALS** PER SERVING

Many people would immediately dismiss choux pastry as too much of an indulgence. However, using low-fat butter and sweetener makes a huge dent in calories. With just a hint of chocolate and squirty cream, these are the ultimate in sweet treats.

Special Occasion

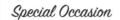

(F)

MAKES 10

2 tbsp granulated sweetener

¼ tsp salt

7 tbsp low-fat butter

½ cup plus 2 tbsp cold water

¾ cup plus 1 tbsp self-raising flour

2 large eggs

2 tbsp dark chocolate chips

10 tbsp reduced-fat whipped cream

Tip

You could bake the pastry buns in advance and freeze them. Simply defrost, fill and serve.

Preheat the oven to 375°F (fan 350°F) and line a baking tray with parchment paper.

Put the sweetener, salt, low-fat butter and water in a saucepan and bring to the boil. As soon as the mixture reaches the boil, take the pan off the heat and gradually beat in the flour. The mixture will look lumpy at first, but persevere. Continue to beat until the mixture forms a ball of dough and comes away from the sides of the saucepan. Add the eggs to the mixture and beat well to incorporate. It will look like the mixture has split at first, but continue to beat until it becomes glossy.

Spoon the mixture into a piping bag fitted with a large nozzle. Pipe ten eclairs onto the lined baking tray (they'll be around 5 in long each). Dab any "tails" down with a wet finger and bake in the oven for 40 minutes. After this time, check and see if the eclairs sound hollow when tapped, are a deep golden colour and crisp. They may need up to 60 minutes depending on your oven. DO NOT OPEN THE OVEN before 40 minutes! Not even for a sneaky peek – they'll likely collapse and you'll end up with pancakes!

Once the time is up, remove the eclairs from the oven and leave to cool on a wire rack. Only fill them when you are ready to serve – aerosol cream doesn't keep its shape very long once squirted! (You can freeze them at this point, prior to filling.)

Once completely cool, cut lengthways through three-quarters of each eclair. Melt the chocolate chips in a bowl in the microwave. Squirt 1 tablespoon of reduced-fat aerosol cream into each split eclair and drizzle the melted chocolate over the tops. Serve immediately.

Bakewell
TARTS

🕐 **10 MINS** | 🍲 **35 MINS** | 💧 **70 CALS** PER SERVING

Everyone loves a bakewell tart. Sweet almond, with tart jam to balance it, makes for a delicious treat that surely can't be slimming friendly. With some clever ingredients, however, this recipe will really surprise you. Authentic flavours minus the guilt – perfection!

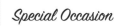

Special Occasion

F

MAKES 10

low-calorie cooking spray
2 low-calorie tortilla wraps
3 tbsp self-raising flour
5 tsp low-fat butter
1 large egg
2 tbsp granulated sweetener
1 tsp almond extract
2 tbsp reduced-sugar raspberry jam
1 tbsp sliced almonds

Preheat the oven to 375°F (fan 350°F) and spray ten holes of a twelve-hole muffin tin with low-calorie cooking spray.

Cut five rounds from each wrap using a 2¾ in pastry cutter to fit the muffin tin. Place each round in a greased muffin tin hole, pushing them into place so they come up the sides of the holes. Bake in the oven for 8 minutes.

Meanwhile, combine the flour, low-fat butter, egg, sweetener and almond extract in a mixing bowl.

Remove the "pastry" shells from the oven and distribute the jam evenly among them, spreading it out a little in the shells.

Spoon a little of the batter into each pastry shell, ensuring the jam is covered by the mix (but avoid overfilling them). Sprinkle the flaked almonds on top and bake in the oven for 25 minutes until golden.

Remove the tin from the oven and allow to cool for a few minutes before removing the tarts from the tin and transferring to a wire rack.

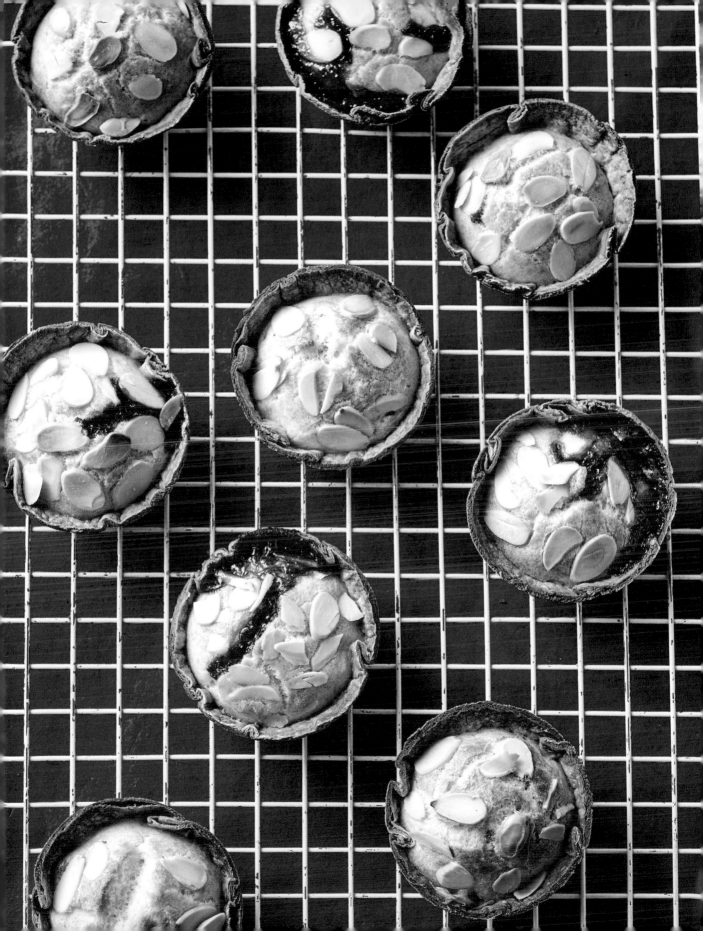

MINI COFFEE
and PECAN CAKES

🕐 **10 MINS** | 🍲 **16 MINS** | 🔥 **50 CALS** PER CAKE

Another one of our "a little of what you fancy" recipes, these lovely mini coffee and pecan cakes will really satisfy any sweet tooth. You won't notice the small ingredient substitutions that make these lower in calories than most cakes. With wonderfully soft sponge and a rich buttercream, these are perfect for parties and special occasions.

— *Special Occasion* —

(F)

MAKES 24

FOR THE CAKES
6 tbsp self-raising flour
3½ tbsp low-fat butter
1 tbsp cocoa powder
2½ tbsp granulated sweetener
pinch of salt
2 large eggs
1 tsp baking powder
1 tbsp instant coffee powder
24 pecan halves, to decorate

FOR THE BUTTERCREAM
1 tsp cocoa powder
5 tsp low-fat butter
½ cup sifted sugar
1 tsp instant coffee powder

Preheat the oven to 375°F (fan 350°F).

Place all of the cake ingredients (except the pecan halves) in a bowl and mix with an electric hand whisk until the mixture is light and smooth.

Place a heaped teaspoon of the cake mixture into each mould of a twenty-four-hole mini silicone muffin tray, dividing the mixture evenly among all twenty-four holes. Transfer to the oven and bake for about 16 minutes until risen and baked through.

Remove the cakes from the oven, then take them out of the tray and leave to cool on a wire rack. (You can freeze the baked cakes when cooled for sandwiching on another day.)

Mix the buttercream ingredients together in a bowl. When the cakes have cooled, slice them in half through the middle. Spread or pipe some buttercream onto one half of the cakes, and place the tops back on. Pop a tiny blob of buttercream on the top of each cake and add a pecan half. Store in an airtight container and keep for up to 3 days.

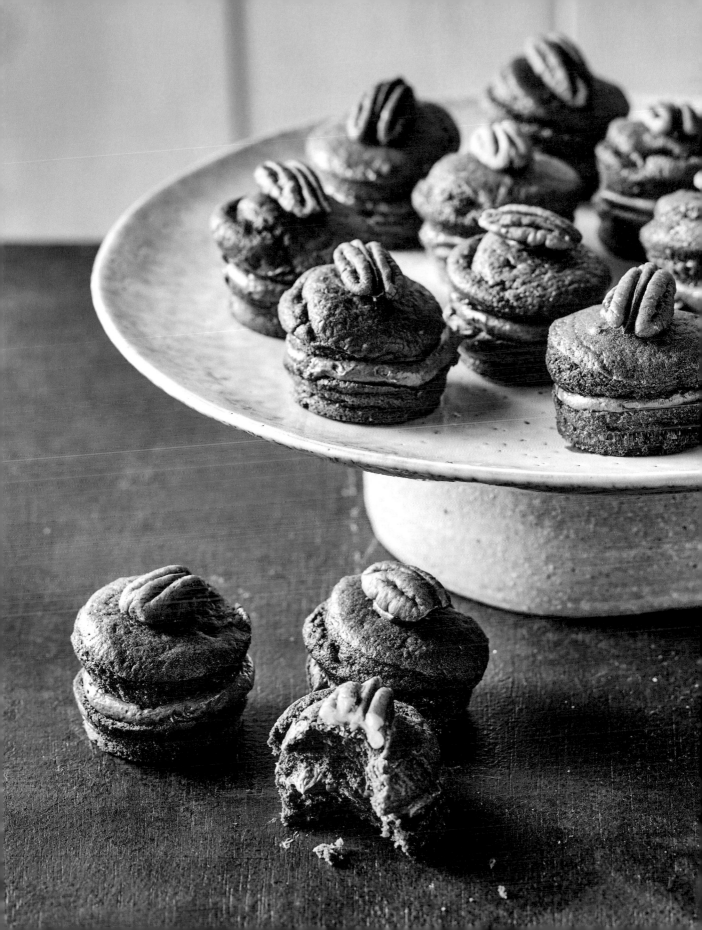

PLUM *and* ALMOND
BREAD PUDDING

🕐 **5 MINS** | 🍲 **10 MINS** | 🔥 **250 CALS** PER SERVING

This recipe is incredibly simple, yet packs a real flavour punch. Using a drop of almond extract and unsweetened almond milk, it is full of natural sweetness. A lighter bread pudding – what more could you want?

Special Occasion

(F)

SERVES 4

¾ cup plus 1 tbsp unsweetened almond milk
½ tsp almond extract
2 tbsp granulated sweetener
2 large eggs
2 slices of white bread, each slice cut into 24 cubes
2 medium plums, halved, stoned and each half cut into 8 slices

Preheat the oven to 375°F (fan 350°F).

Heat the almond milk in a pan over a low heat but do not let it boil. Add the almond extract and 1 tbsp of the sweetener.

Whisk the eggs in a medium bowl, then whisk in the warmed milk.

If you're using 4 in ovenproof ramekins, place six cubes of bread in the bottom of each one. Top with six slices of plum, sprinkle each with half a teaspoon of sweetener, then place another six cubes of bread on top.

Divide the egg mix equally among the four dishes, top each one with two slices of plum, and sprinkle with the remaining sweetener. Allow to stand for 5 minutes so the bread can absorb the custard. (Alternatively you could layer each ingredient in one 9 in ovenproof dish.)

Place the ramekins or baking dish on a baking tray. (You can freeze the pudding at this point for cooking on another day.)

Cook for 10 minutes or until the egg has set and the top is golden, then serve.

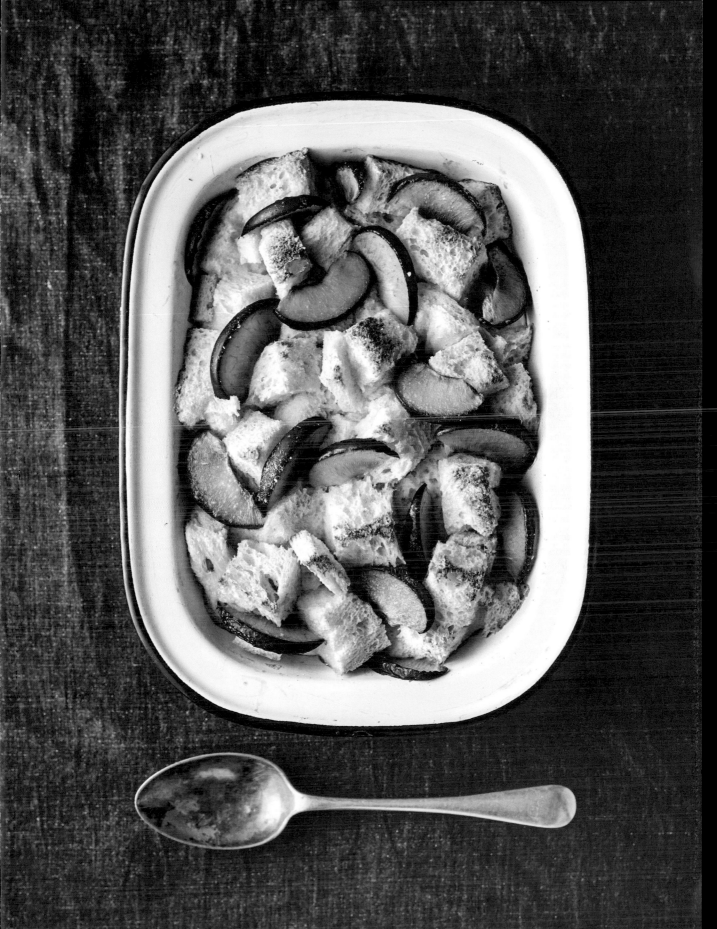

Salted Caramel
BANOFFEE PIES

🕐 **20 MINS** │ 🍲 **NO COOK** │ 🔥 **234 CALS** PER SERVING

Making banoffee pie slimming friendly was a mission we took very seriously!
There's no room to compromise on that distinctive taste. This version makes
a few simple ingredient swaps to reduce the calories, but what about the
flavour? It's bang on! We love serving this dessert for dinner parties, but we
have to admit to throwing it together for a weeknight treat, too.

―――――――――――――― *Special Occasion* ――――――――――――――

SERVES 4

2 tsp low-fat butter
8 Lotus Biscoff biscuits
   (or other caramelized biscuits)
7 tbsp low-fat cream cheese
¾ cup fat-free Greek-style yogurt
3 tbsp granulated sweetener
2 tsp salted caramel flavouring
2 bananas
1 tsp lemon juice
1 tbsp salted caramel sauce

Melt the low-fat butter in a bowl in the microwave for around
10 seconds.

Crush the Lotus Biscoff biscuits into fine crumbs in a bowl. Pour
over the melted low-fat butter and mix to combine fully. Divide
the biscuit mixture among four ramekins and press it down
firmly into each dish. Pop the ramekins in the fridge for
10 minutes to allow the biscuit base to firm up.

Meanwhile, mix the light cream cheese, Greek yogurt,
sweetener and salted caramel flavouring in a bowl until smooth.
Place in the fridge until the pies are ready to assemble.

Peel and cut the bananas into thin slices. Place them in a bowl
and coat them with the lemon juice – this will stop the banana
from discolouring.

Remove the ramekins from the fridge and add a layer of
banana slices on top of the biscuit base. Spoon the chilled
cheesecake mix on top of the banana layer, then finish with
another layer of banana slices.

Drizzle over the salted caramel sauce and serve.

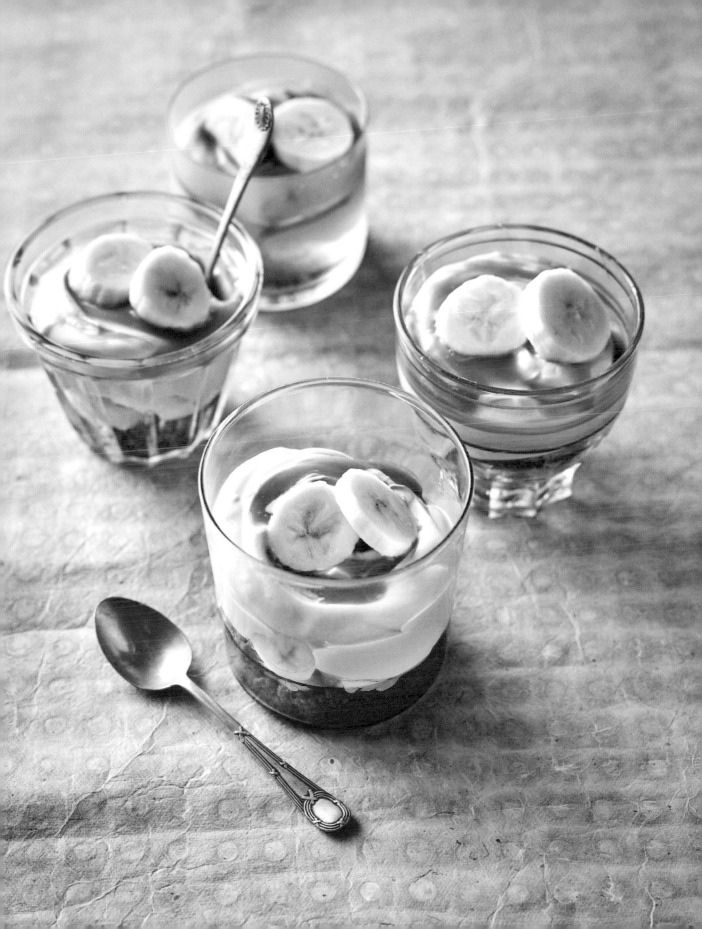

STICKY TOFFEE
Pudding

🕐 **5 MINS** | 🍲 **20 MINS** | 🔥 **233 CALS** PER SERVING

We know what you're thinking: a sticky toffee pudding in a slimming book? At Pinch of Nom, our determination to make slimming-friendly desserts is real. This sticky toffee pudding is definitely a winner. Sweet and luxuriously indulgent, you won't believe the low calorie count!

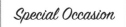

Special Occasion

F

SERVES 4

low-calorie cooking spray
9 tbsp self-raising flour
1 tsp baking powder
1 tbsp molasses
3 tbsp granulated sweetener
3½ tbsp low-fat butter
3 medium eggs
1 tbsp golden syrup

Preheat the oven to 375°F (fan 350°F) and spray four ovenproof ramekins with low-calorie cooking spray.

Put all of the ingredients in a large mixing bowl (except the golden syrup) and whisk with an electric hand whisk until fully combined, light and airy.

Distribute the golden syrup evenly among the ramekins. Top with the cake mixture and bake in the oven for about 20 minutes until just cooked through.

Remove from the oven and leave to cool slightly in the ramekins, then turn out into serving dishes. Serve with golden syrup or your choice of accompaniment.

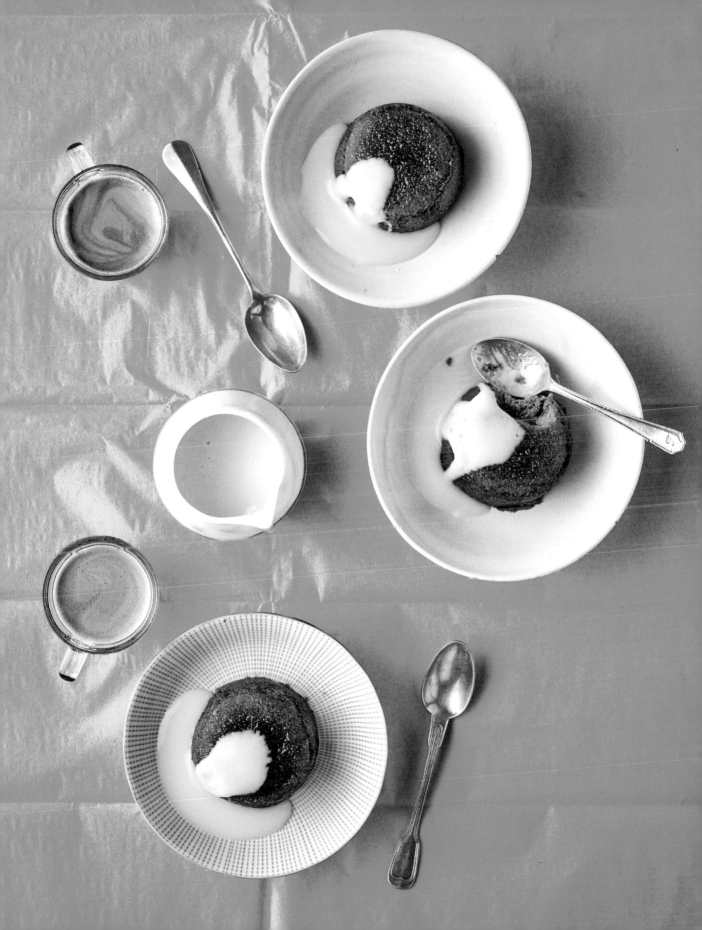

Crème **BRULEE**

🕐 **5 MINS** | 📦 **35 MINS** | 🔥 **279 CALS** PER SERVING

It's hard to believe a crème brûlée could make it into this book, but here it is and it's an absolute treat of a recipe. By swapping a few of the classic ingredients you can save on calories while not compromising on the taste. This will become a firm favourite for dinner parties or school nights – a dessert you can enjoy without any fear of overindulging.

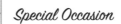

———————— _Special Occasion_ ————————

SERVES 6

1⅔ cups skim milk
2 large eggs plus 2 large egg yolks
2 tsp vanilla paste or extract
4 tbsp granulated sweetener
6 tsp superfine sugar

Preheat the oven to 375°F (fan 350°F) and place six ovenproof ramekins in a large, deep baking dish.

Put the milk, eggs and yolks, vanilla and sweetener in a large jug and mix really well – you're not trying to whisk any air into the mixture so just mix it gently with a fork until all the egg is fully combined.

Divide the mixture evenly among the ramekins, then carefully fill the baking dish with boiling water until it reaches about halfway up the sides of the ramekins. Place in the oven and cook for 35 minutes, or until the egg mixture is set.

Remove from the oven, take out of the baking dish and leave to cool.

Once cool, sprinkle a teaspoon of caster sugar onto each crème brûlée and shake gently so the sugar covers the top. Melt the sugar with a blowtorch, then wait for the sugar to harden and form a crunchy top before serving. If using a broiler, make sure it is really hot, place the crème brûlée as close to the broiler as possible and watch very closely to make sure the sugar doesn't burn – again, leave to cool and let the sugar set before serving.

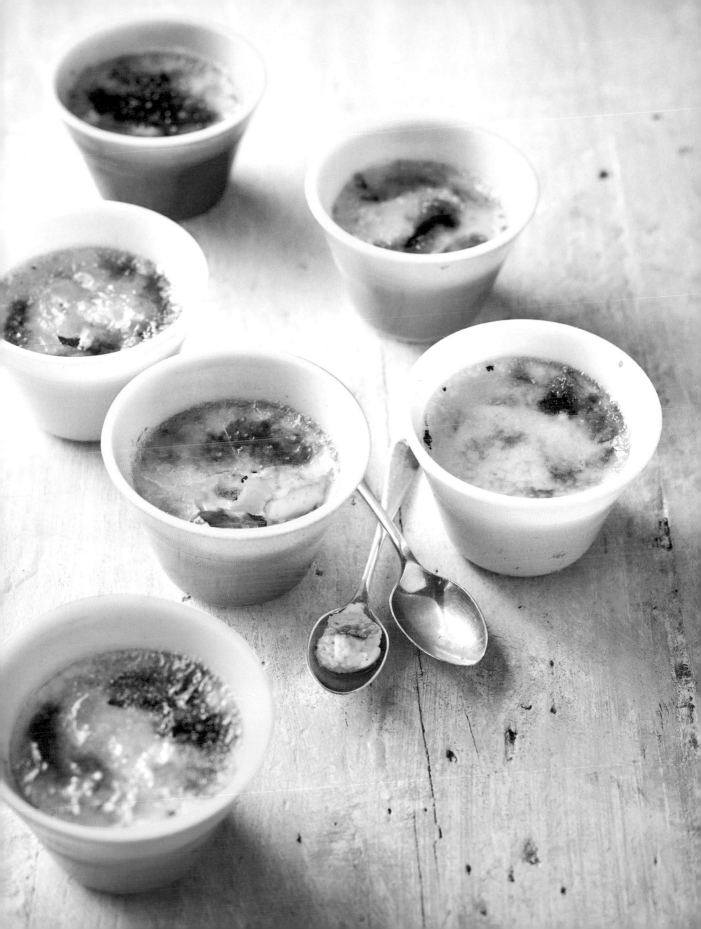

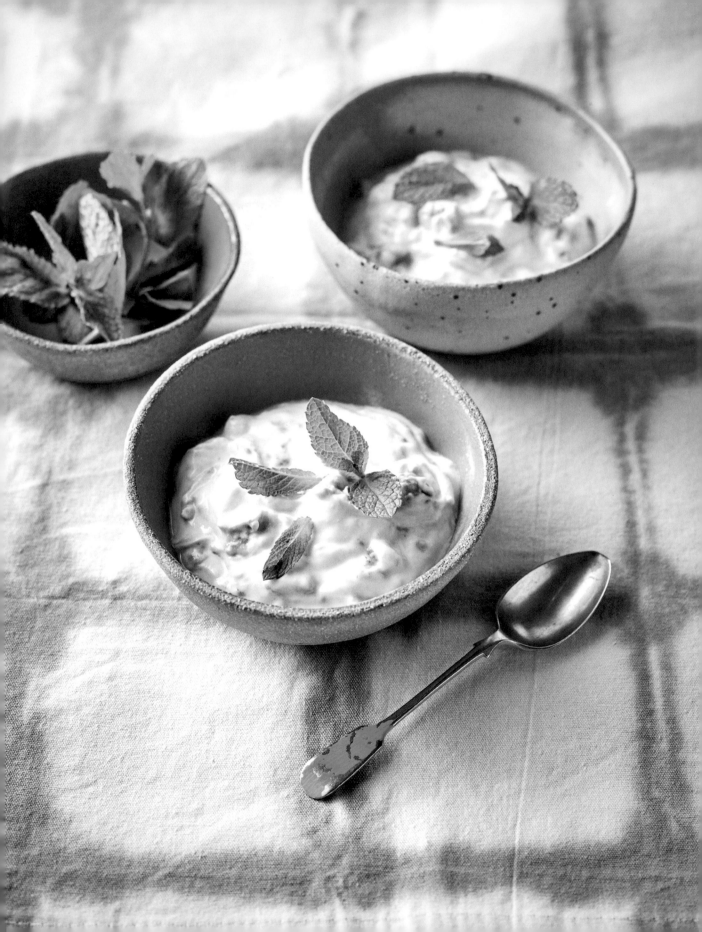

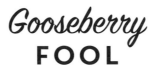

Gooseberry
FOOL

🕙 **10 MINS** (PLUS CHILLING TIME) | 🍲 **10 MINS** | 🔥 **249 CALS** PER SERVING

Sharp and sweet at the same time, gooseberries are perfect for a good, creamy fool. And "fool" is a fantastic name for these as they will fool you into thinking they are heavy with cream. Instead, this recipe uses quark, an unflavoured soft cheese which gives a rich creaminess to dishes while being low in fat.

--- *Special Occasion* ---

GF

SERVES 2

7 oz gooseberries
2 tbsp plus 2 tsp granulated
   sweetener
½ cup quark (or more yogurt)
½ cup fat-free Greek-style yogurt
2 tsp sugar-free elderflower cordial
mint leaves, to serve (optional)

Place the gooseberries in a saucepan, cover and cook over a low heat for about 10 minutes, until they soften and start to fall apart. Remove from the heat, stir in the 2 tablespoons of sweetener and leave to cool.

Whisk together the quark and yogurt in a bowl until combined, then stir in the cooled gooseberries, elderflower cordial and the remaining 2 teaspoons of sweetener. Place in the fridge for 30 minutes, then divide between two bowls and serve garnished with mint, if you like.

APPLE STRUDEL

🕐 **10 MINS** | 🗑 **10 MINS** | 🔥 **278 CALS** PER SERVING

When we first put this recipe up on the website, it caused quite a stir. So much so that a leading brand of tortilla wraps actually sold out! Luckily, they're back in stock, alongside other brands of low-calorie tortilla wraps, meaning you can get that beautiful pastry-like texture and taste, minus the calories.

Special Occasion

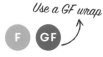

Use a GF wrap

F GF

SERVES 1

1 baking apple, peeled and chopped

½ tsp ground cinnamon

2 tsp granulated sweetener, plus extra for sprinkling

1 tbsp water

2 tsp mincemeat – check it is vegetarian

1 low-calorie tortilla wrap

1 medium egg, beaten

low-calorie cooking spray

Stir the apple, cinnamon, sweetener and water in a microwaveable bowl. Cover with cling film and cook on high for 2 minutes or until the apple starts to soften but still has bite.

Drain off any excess water from the bowl then measure out ¼ cup of cooked apple to mix through the mincemeat. (Save the rest for another day.)

Preheat the oven to 400°F (fan 375°F). The next stages are a bit tricky, so there are some visual steps overleaf.

Fold the wrap into three equal sections. Press firmly so you can see the marks when you unfold it. Open out the wrap and fold it in half vertically. You should be able to see all the fold lines.

Using a sharp knife, make a diagonal cut about two fingers' width from the bottom of the wrap, running from the fold line to the edge of the wrap. Measure another finger's width and make another cut at the same angle. Continue cutting (you should get 6–8 strips), leaving the top and bottom of the wrap uncut.

Open out the wrap and brush the whole thing with beaten egg, paying extra attention to the edges. Spoon the apple mixture along the middle of the wrap. Fold the top and bottom of the wrap in, then starting at the end closest to you, fold the bottom left strip up towards the top right-hand corner of the wrap. Fold the bottom right strip over towards the top left corner of the wrap. Alternate the remaining strips until all the filling is enclosed. Sprinkle with a little sweetener.

Spray a baking tray with low-calorie cooking spray, put the filled wrap on the tray and bake in the oven for 10 minutes or until golden brown. Remove from the oven and enjoy warm.

Tip

You can freeze the apple strudel parcels before they go into the oven. Simply defrost before baking as normal.

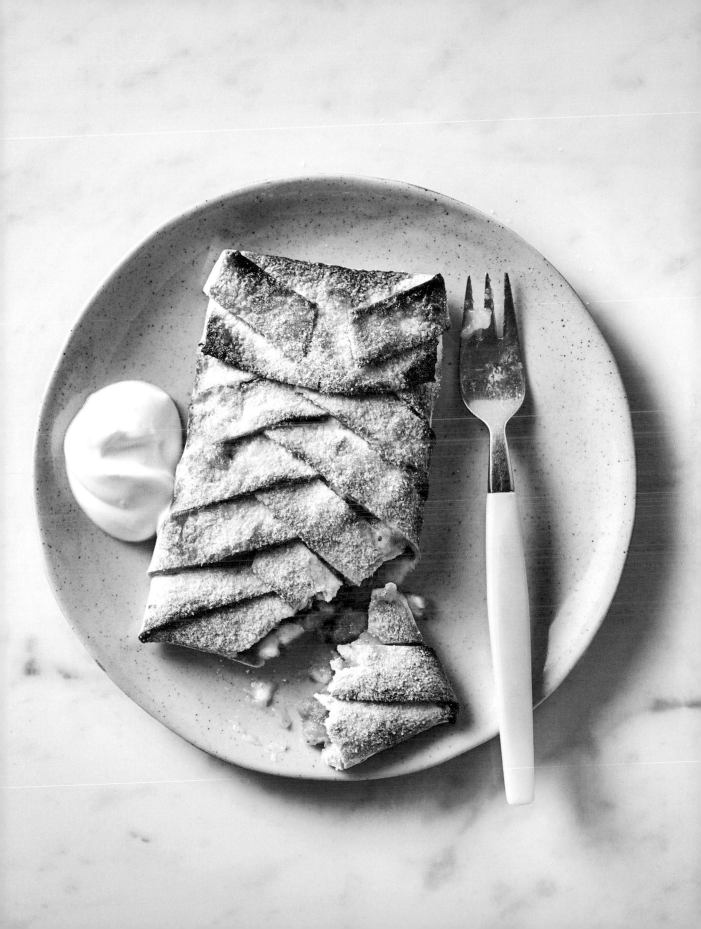

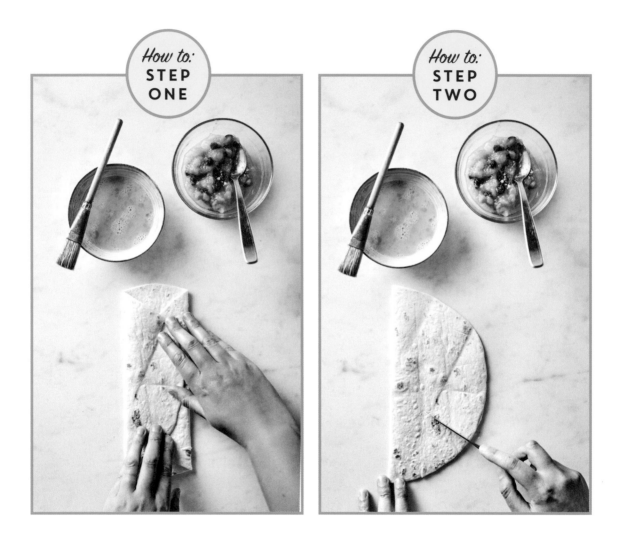

How to:
**STEP
ONE**

How to:
**STEP
TWO**

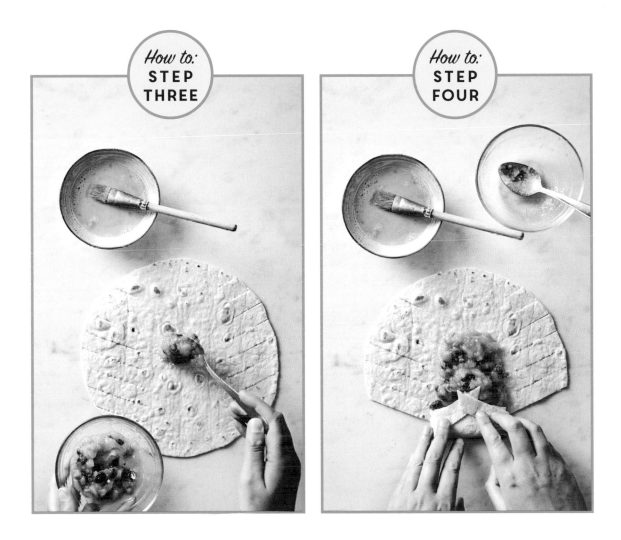

How to:
STEP
THREE

How to:
STEP
FOUR

Pina Colada
BAKED RICE PUDDING

🕐 **5 MINS** | 🍲 **1 HOUR 45 MINS** | 🔥 **298 CALS** PER SERVING

This may seem like an odd combination, until you realize that the flavours of coconut and pineapple are made for each other! This warming and decadent-tasting rice pudding will amaze you with its low calorie content. So creamy, so good; it is the sort of recipe we dream of when following a diet.

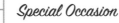 *Special Occasion*

SERVES 2

low-calorie cooking spray
heaping ½ cup Arborio risotto rice
2 tsp granulated sweetener
2½ cups coconut milk (or other dairy alternative)
⅔ cup pineapple chunks
grated zest of 1 lime

Preheat the oven to 350°F (fan 325°F) and spray a 6 in ovenproof dish with low-calorie cooking spray.

Add the rice, sweetener and coconut milk to the dish and stir well to dissolve the sweetener. Cover with foil and bake in the oven for 1 hour 45 minutes.

Mix the pineapple in a bowl with the lime zest.

Remove the pudding from the oven. (You can allow the pudding to cool, then cover and freeze at this point for reheating on another day.)

When ready to serve, spoon it into two bowls and top with the pineapple.

Tip
Why not add a splash of rum to the pineapple topping for an extra-special treat?

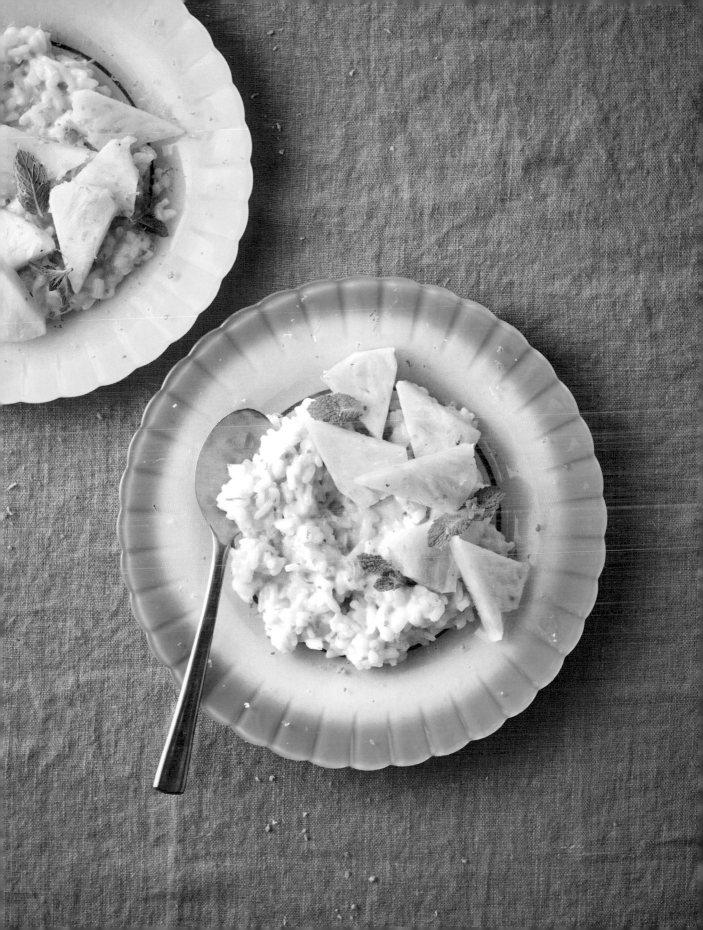

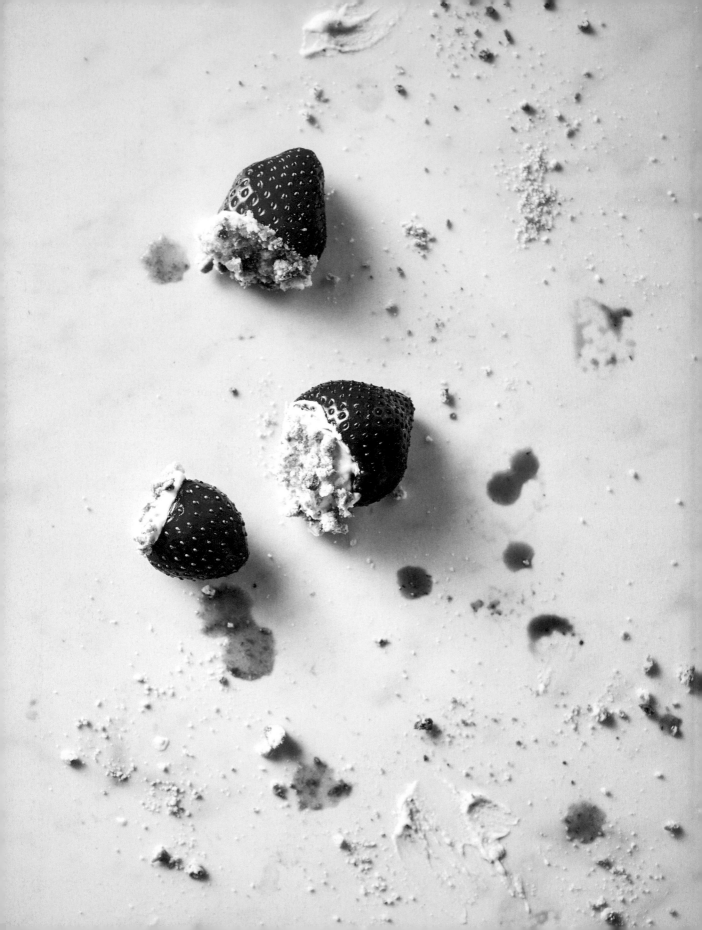

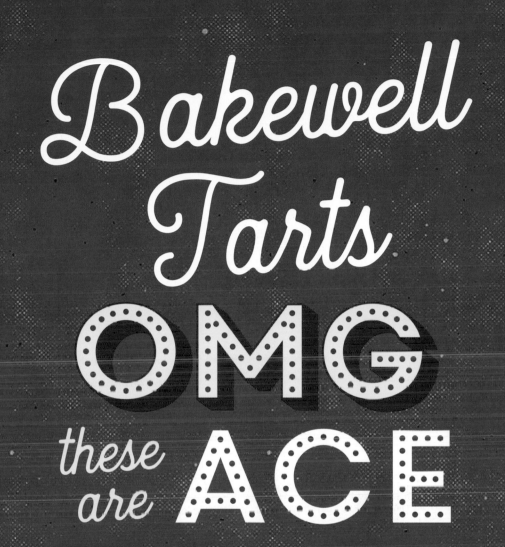

Bakewell Tarts **OMG** these are **ACE**

GAYLE

"

The **STICKY TOFFEE PUDDING** is even nicer than the puddings you get in the supermarket – *delicious!*

LAURA

The **CHOCOLATE ECLAIRS** were a *huge hit* with everyone. My 13-year-old said they are better than store-bought.

DONNA

INDEX

ACKNOWLEDGMENTS

Writing a book is harder than we ever could have imagined and wouldn't have been possible without the help of so many wonderful people. Firstly we want to say a huge thank you to all of our followers on social media and all those who make our recipes. Without you, this book just wouldn't have been possible. We're so proud that Pinch of Nom has helped so many people.

Thank you to our publisher Carole and to Martha and the rest of the team at Bluebird for helping us create this book. It's been a fun, exciting and amazing journey seeing this book come to life.

To Mike for the bangin' photos and to Kate for making things look so amazing. Thanks also to Flossy for all your help in the process. Thanks to Emma for the brilliant design.

We also want to thank our friends and family who made this book possible. Special thanks go to Laura, Emma and Lisa for the endless hours you've put into this and for putting up with us driving you round the bend! Additional thanks go to Meadows, Janie and Vince. Thanks to all of you for making Nom work and for keeping everything ticking over. We're so proud to work with you lot.

To Jackie, Teresa, Tracy, Emma B, Cheryl, Little Laura, Jill, Michelle, Shelley, Rebecca, thank you for taking care of our Facebook group. We'd also like to say thank you to each and every member of our Facebook group. From sharing stories, thoughts and ideas, to sharing transformation pictures and personal successes, you've believed in Pinch of Nom from day one and we can't thank you enough that all of your support has meant we've been able to do this book.

Our thanks also to our amazing taste testing group for all your help in sending feedback and suggestions for these recipes. We have really appreciated the time you gave to support this project.

To Boris, Dima and Leo for teaching us all that we know. Our agent Clare for believing in us from day one. And to Sue, Paula and Jo – without your inspiration we wouldn't be here.

And finally … huge thanks go to Cath and Paul for all of your support, and for letting us take over your kitchen to create all of these recipes.

ABOUT THE AUTHORS

KATE *and* KAY

Founders of Pinch of Nom
www.pinchofnom.com

Kate Allinson and Kay Featherstone owned a restaurant together on the Wirral, where Kate was head chef. Together they created the Pinch of Nom blog with the aim of teaching people how to cook. They began sharing healthy, slimming recipes and today Pinch of Nom is the UK's most visited food blog with an active and engaged online community of over 1.5 million followers.

THANKS TO ALL THE PINCH OF NOM TASTE TESTERS

HANNAH DURANT · Shannon HARRIMAN · CHARLENE SHARMAN · NIAMH ANNE · LENA DENT · JANET LEE

LUCI VINŠOVÁ · SAMMIE BULLIMORE · STEPHANIE CONNELLY · RACHEL HOARE · LAURA JOHNSON · Michelle JACKSON

LIZ LEVIS · HANNAH MORRISON · Diane RITCHIE · DEIRDRE COOKE · Nicola MAYREN · JIM FORD

Simone KELLY · KRISTINA INGRAM · NATALIE HILSTON-THÉVENOT · Jade BRANDWOOD · LYNSEY ROBINSON · JUDITH HUNTER

MANDY SMITH · EMMA MANNERS-LILLEY · VIVIAN DAVIDSON · Nicola GREEN · KATY BROWN · ROBYN DICKSON

Vienna TAYLOR · EILEEN MURPHY BINGHAM · KERRY MARVELL · Helen Pettit · LINDA HENDERSON · Natalie CHAPMAN

HEATHER PARKER · LINDA HEDLEY · Catriona DEACON · RHIANNON DASHFIELD · LISA ORETO · Louise WRIGHT

VICTORIA PRIESTLEY · Charlee CHOREMI · GILLIAN KENNEDY · Natalie GIBSON · AMANDA CAMERON · KATRINA CANN

Jennifer Edwards · MICHELLE WHITTEN · LEYLA PATTISON · KEELA DARBY · Jazmin WEBSTER · RIA TONGE

JULIE SWAYZE · Karen PEARSON · Demi HICKS · KATHRYN READ · ANGELA HARRISON · Denise BINNIE

Charles SWYER · Tara BROWN · NATHAN WINFIELD · LAURA CLIFFORDE · MARK BIRCH · Anita Sanderman

BRIAN HOPCROFT · Joanne HUDDART · JENNY DEVLIN · JULIA HARRIS · Caitlin WALTON · LYNN HARGREAVES-MCCALLUM

ALYSSA ANKRAH · NATALIE LAVERY · Celine-Anne SEARLE · BECKY WRIGLEY · Emma-Jane DEAN · SARAH PICKERSGILL

LAUREN NAPIER · ANITA PRIOR · PAULA GLASBEY · BECCA MILLS · CAROLINE YORKE · Sophie HUCKSTEP

Joanne LARDER · Emma HOPE · Nicole-Alix DEVLIN · Kim Youngman · CLAIRE DAW · MEGAN O'TODD